YOU
ON A
DIET

Also by Michael F. Roizen and Mehmet C. Oz
YOU: Staying Young

Also by Michael F. Roizen
RealAge: Are You as Young as You Can Be?

YOU
ON A
DIET

Lose up to 2 inches from your waist in 2 weeks

MICHAEL F. ROIZEN, MD
MEHMET C. OZ, MD

Authors of the million-copy bestselling
You: The Owner's Manual

WITH TED SPIKER; LISA OZ AND CRAIG WYNETT
ILLUSTRATIONS BY GARY HALLGREN

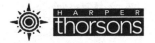

HarperThorsons
An Imprint of HarperCollins*Publishers*
77–85 Fulham Palace Road,
Hammersmith, London W6 8JB

The website address is: www.thorsonselement.com

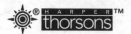

and *HarperThorsons* are trademarks of
HarperCollins*Publishers* Ltd

First published in the US by Free Press,
a division of Simon & Schuster, Inc 2006
First published in the UK by HarperThorsons 2007
This edition 2008

1 3 5 7 9 10 8 6 4 2

A catalogue record of this book is
available from the British Library

ISBN-13 978-0-00-726440-7
ISBN-10 0-00-726440-2

Printed and bound in Great Britain by
Clays Ltd, St Ives plc

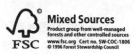

To the millions who have dieted hard,
so they can learn to diet smart

DISCLAIMER

CONTENTS

PART I

WHAT A WAIST!

How your body is supposed to look –
and work

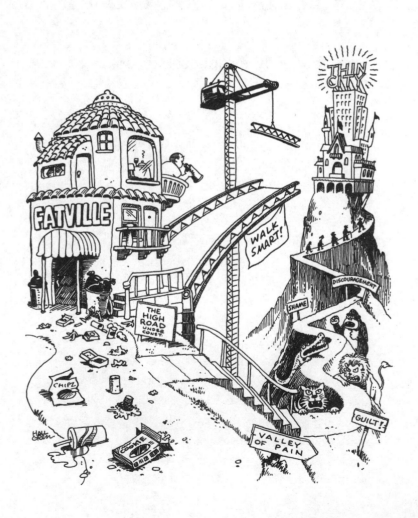

YOU: ON A DIET

Work smarter, not harder

Most diets promise common sense solutions to tight-waistband problems: eat less, and you'll weigh less. Keep your mouth closed, and you'll keep the pounds off. Sweat like a sauna-dwelling sumo wrestler, and you'll end up skinnier than a sheet of paper. Straight-forward enough. But if it really worked that way, our bodies wouldn't be large enough to be spotted by Google Earth. If it really worked that way, then most diets wouldn't fail.

Or it could be that most diets have it all wrong.

We believe it's the latter.

You know why? Because most diets instruct you to take on the chips, pizzas and cakes with brute force. It's you versus food in a lifetime heavyweight fight. But in that scenario, the fight is always fixed – and not in your favour. That's because the battle against extra pounds isn't won with force, with sweat, with *trying* to diet. It's won with elegance, with smart and healthy choices that become as automatic as a Simon Cowell barb.

When it comes to dieting, trying to whip fat with our weapon of willpower is the food equivalent of holding your breath under water. You can do it for a while, but no matter how psyched up you get, at some point your body – your biology – forces you to the surface gasping for air. And with most diets, your body forces you to gasp (or gulp) for food. No matter how hard you try not to eat, some hidden force deep inside is always prising your mouth back open, making it impossible for willpower to win. Instead of sparring with your waistline, it's time you made your body an ally in the fight against fat.

Our process is to look at our overweight bodies the way scientists would: identify the underlying biology of the problem, then find the cures. Why? Because we're lucky enough to be in the right place at the right time – a time when the scientific world has just started to unlock the biological mysteries that have caused us to store fat and gain weight. By making this knowledge simple and accessible, we're going to give you tools and actions to crack the code of true and lifelong waist management. In fact, our plan will help you avoid the dangerous yo-yo cycle of weight gain and weight loss. We're going to help you reprogram your body so that you can keep off the weight you lose forever.

Through the years, many of us have been led to believe that our weight problem is about two things: calorie counting and mental toughness. While some of us may say that the weight problem is down to too much lasagne, the real problem is that most of us have as much of a clue about how our bodies work as we have about how our cars do. Yes, we know the major parts and generally what they're supposed to do. But, if we look under our bonnet, do we really understand the systems that make our bodies accelerate to a life of fat and the ones that slam the brake on the dangerous biscuit-and-cake collisions that take place every day? Probably not, and that's what we're here to help you learn.

Above all, we're going to teach you that when it comes to dieting, you need to work smart, not hard.

Following our plan, you can expect to drop up to two inches from your waist (or a dress size) within two weeks and see results steadily after that. While the end goal is what many of us look for, we believe that the path you choose to get there is what really dictates whether you make it or not.

As we travel through the book, you'll notice various ways you'll learn about your body and how to change it. These are the five main elements we'll use along the way:

YOU-reka Moments: Like Einstein suddenly realizing that $E = mc^2$ you'll develop deep insights that challenge your preconceptions about diets, fat and your body.

YOUR Body: In Parts II and III, we'll start each chapter by giving quick biology lessons about what really happens inside your body. We believe that by learning about how the inside of your body works, you'll develop the knowledge you need to change how the outside looks.

YOU Tests: Through interactive quizzes and measurements, you'll establish baselines for such vital statistics as your ideal body size and your eating personality. And you'll also be able to test for the secret things that could be contributing to a weight problem (see our tongue test on page 67).

YOU Tips: After we explore the biology of your body to show you what bad things can happen if you make the wrong choice or have cross-wired genetics, we'll immediately give you actions that can help turn your body around. At the end of each chapter, we'll outline intelligent strategies – big and small – for living, eating and moving in a healthier way.

The YOU Diet and Activity Plan: In Part IV (on page 205) we'll detail the specific and simple strategies, recipes and exercises that will lead you to the body you want – for the rest of your life. The 14-day YOU Diet (it's actually so easy that we crafted a seven-day plan that you do twice) and the no-weights-required YOU Workout provide all the tools and instructions you'll need. Best of all, they don't take a lot of time, and they're so easy that you can incorporate them into your life today.

So where do we start? With our first YOU-reka! moment:

YOU-reka!
Your body naturally wants to take you to your optimum weight, as long as you don't get in its way.

That's right. For almost everyone, no matter what your genetics, the systems, organs and processes of your body all want you to function at an ideal weight and size. With the following few principles that we'll develop throughout the book, we're going to teach you how you can make that happen without having to bludgeon yourself in frustration with a butter knife. These are our major principles of achieving your very best and healthiest body.

YOU Will Choose Elegance over Force

Most dieters try to defeat their cream cake infatuations with will, with deprivation, with sweat, with a 'my-brain-is-stronger-than-your-crust' attitude. But trying to beat your body with mind power alone may be more painful than passing a melon-size kidney stone. Instead, you have to learn about the systems and actions that influence hunger, satiety, fat storing and fat burning to fine-tune your corporeal vehicle so it runs on autopilot and takes you to your ultimate destination: a healthy, ideal body. (For those who want to skip ahead, you've probably already peeked at Part IV; however, getting to know the nuances of your body is what will help you achieve and maintain a truly healthy-size body.)

FACTOID

When you lose weight without exercise, you lose both muscle and fat, but when you gain weight without exercise, you gain only fat. It's much easier to gain fat weight than it is to gain muscle weight, which is one of the reasons why yo-yo dieting fails so miserably: When you continually gain and lose and gain and lose, you end up gaining proportionally even more fat, because of the muscle loss that takes place every time you lose.

YOU Will Learn How Your Body Thinks

True body improvement is about science. The only way you'll understand the way calories and fat travel from that 2,000-calorie pizza to the back of your arm is by bringing alive the physiology of hormones, blood, organs and muscles – by explaining the processes of digestion, starvation, fat storage and muscle movements. Just as when you're trying to help a tantruming toddler or kick-start a frozen computer, you can't fix it unless you know what's wrong. Know the *why*, and it's much easier to handle the *how* – when you need to. Let's face it, we're not going to be sitting next to you at 10.30pm when you're pilfering a doughnut. So you need to be equipped with knowledge of how your body works and reacts to that doughnut so that you can defend against the little sugar-coated bugger.

YOU Will Challenge Your Beliefs about Diets

Throughout our lives, we've been conditioned to believe that if one thing is good for us, then more of it must be better. If you eliminate 100 calories from your daily diet, then eliminating 400 must qualify you for size 8. If you walk to lose weight, then running a marathon must nuke the fat right off your body. Well, neither idea is true. Worse, not only aren't they true, but many of the diet myths perpetuated today actually *hurt* our bodies. Food deprivation, for example, drops your metabolism and makes your body want to *store* fat.

In a way, we live on the two extremes of a pendulum. Either we swing all the way in one direction (strict, tedious dieting with a draconian low daily calorie intake), or we swing all the way in the other direction (stuffing ourselves with rubbish). We have to stop swinging so much and start living in the middle of that pendulum by striking a balance and avoiding the periods of extreme 'ons' and 'offs'.

One of the reasons why most so-called diets fail is because of a psychological and behavioural flaw that many dieters have. We desperately want to believe the simple, comforting promises that diets make – that doing A always gets us B. Because once we see that A (eating wheat germ 24/7) doesn't always equal B (the cover of *Vogue*), then we get frustrated and angry, and give in to the gods of cream-filled baked goods.

Unfortunately, your body and your fat do not have a linear, two-step relationship. Instead, think of your body as an orchestra. All of its systems, organs, muscles, cells, fluids, hormones and chemicals play different instruments, make different sounds (your intestines play in the tuba section), and produce different results depending on how you use them. They work independently, but only when they're played together can you appreciate the magnificent symphony of your own biology. As the conductor of your biological orchestra, you control how the instruments interact and what the final result will be.

YOU Will Make Dieting Automatic

While we want you to 'not think' about eating good foods, we also know that 'not thinking' may be how you got into this waistband-stretching mess in the first place. When you don't think about the consequences of ordering football-size pizzas, you end up with such pleasantries as high LDL (bad) cholesterol, low HDL (healthy type of) cholesterol, inflammation in your arteries, and a higher risk of aging arteries that cause memory loss, heart disease, even wrinkles, as well as a steady stream of coupon offers from the large men's department. We want your body to guide you to the *right* choices – without thinking about them – so that they'll lead to the results you want. It will take some effort at the start to retrain your habits, palate and muscles, but this programme will serve as a lifelong eating, activity and behaviour plan that will become as routine as going to the toilet before bed.

Unless you're the rare kind of person who responds to dietary drill sergeants, you won't find long-term solutions using traditional weight-loss methods: willpower, deprivation, fads, phases or dead-bolting the lid of the peanut butter. Instead, using this plan, you will train yourself to *never* think about how much you're eating, *never* think about getting on a diet or worry about coming off one, and *never* have to figure out formulas, zones or, for the love of (fill in the deity of your choice), place a chicken breast on a food scale.

YOU Will Focus on Waist Management

Our society seems almost as obsessed with pounds as it is with celebrity breakups, but it's time to shift your thinking: Studies have shown that waist circumference, not overall weight, is the most important indicator of mortality related to being overweight. Of course you'll lose pounds on this plan, but we want you to switch your focus from a number that measures your *weight* to one that measures your *waist*. Because of its proximity to your organs, your belly fat is the most dangerous fat you can carry.

In addition to helping you shrink your waist through diet, we'll also teach you the exercises that will help you achieve and maintain a healthy waist size. Now, we don't want you to think that exercise must involve sweating like a waterfall and panting like an obscene caller, because it doesn't. But you do need to start thinking about your body as a dartboard: it's all about what's in the centre. You'll be focusing on the physical activities that will help control your waist size – specifically walking and foundation-muscle training of your entire body (without growing igloo-size muscles). We'll teach you simple moves that will develop all of your foundation muscles, and we'll teach you how to tighten your belly, improve your posture and develop the muscles that will make you fit into your clothes better. That translates into a shapelier waist, which, studies show, makes you more attractive to others.

But let's not overlook the management part of the waist-management equation. We all know how good managers work: they plan ahead and create systems that play to people's strengths, they set realistic goals, they measure progress, and they don't force their employees down roads that are designed to give them a pack-your-things meeting with HR. You need to train yourself to be a good waist manager by following a plan that's designed to help you become the CEO of your body.

YOU Test: Take out the Tape

Some people haven't stepped on a scale for years. And that's a good thing. For our purposes, you don't need to know how much you weigh (but if you want to check your progress on this programme, then go ahead and peek). All you need is a tape measure. Measure the circumference of your waist at the point of your belly button, and record the score here. (Depending on how your weight is distributed, you may need to make an adjustment to where you place the tape. If you're obese, keep the tape measure parallel to the floor during measurement.)

YOUR SIZE: _____

For optimum health, the ideal waist size for women is 32½ inches; once you hit 37 inches, the dangers to your health increase. For men, the ideal is 35 inches, and the dangers to your health increase once you hit 40 inches.

While we're going to emphasize waist over weight in this book, we also know that many of you won't be able to resist the siren of the scale. When it comes to actual weight, you do need to stop thinking about one specific number ('I want to get down to nine stone'). All of us have an ideal playing weight – not a weight for running marathons or posing for an airbrushed-anyway centrefold. This ideal playing weight is a *range* in which you live lean and healthy, and one in which you significantly reduce the risks of aging diseases associated with being overweight (more on all of this in Part II).

YOU Will *Focus* on YOU, but Not *Rely* on YOU

It's clear that we all have different builds, just as we all have different genetics, metabolic rates and chemical interactions. Still, there are some fundamental biological facts that are true whether you're built like a branch or a stump. As a species, we're programmed to gain and preserve the right amount of weight. That's simply what our bodies are designed to do (more on that coming up). The trick is to work out your factory settings. Then, we'll give you the all-important tools that will help you to reboot those factory settings so that your body maintains its ideal size and shape.

While this is a very individual challenge, it doesn't have to be a lonely one. Life is a team game, and of course you have the ultimate team: your family. The most successful teams all work in the same way: everybody plays a different role and contributes in their own way. The team can't win the title unless everybody, not just the stars, works for the team goal.

Somehow, though, when it comes to weight control, you believe that you're solely responsible for dropping your excess pounds and changing your habits. To make it worse, it seems that the world is against us in the form of big portions, junk food and family dinners that could feed a small municipality. You have to stop thinking that this game is you versus a stadium full of curry-loving opponents. You won't achieve success without a team that can encourage you when you're doing well, and give you an encouraging kick up the backside when you're not. Your starting lineup should include your doctor, maybe a nutritionist, maybe a personal trainer, and certainly lots of fans like your family and friends (online or in person) who can push you, support you and yank the tube of Pringles away from you. You should also use this opportunity to find a support partner who needs you as much as you need her. After all, the best kinds of satisfaction shouldn't come from the sixth spoonful of ice cream, but from sharing knowledge and support, and helping others lose inches.

YOU Will Stop Blaming Yourself

The classic psychology of fat is this: if you're thin, then you believe that fat people must be doing something wrong to make them fat. But if you're fat, then you blame the environment, your genetics or anything else. Well, we're going to try to eliminate that blame and use medical insights to explain the epic saga of weight-related problems. We want to move dieting past a guilt-driven and blame-ridden system, and make it a science-based system.

Of course, not everyone can look like Cameron Diaz or Brad Pitt. To get an idea of what your healthy weight, waist and shape should be, you'll need to take into account such things as bone structure, muscle mass, genetics and risk factors associated with your weight. Here's a fact that goes virtually unmentioned: there are clinically obese people who live with no risk of health problems, and there are CD-thin people whose risk of dying prematurely is more than a chuteless skydiver's. Our goal is to get you to the point where you strip away inches, you strip away the risks of being overweight, and you strip away the guilt associated with the process of always trying to do so.

YOU Will Never Be Hungry

We know exactly how you've felt when you've dieted in the past. Hungry. Famished. Three seconds away from steamrolling through a bowl of ice cream with sprinkles. That recipe for dieting is one you can tear up. In fact, the only place hunger ever got you was a pair of trousers that could double as curtains. To eat and work smart, your goal is *never* to be hungry and *never* to be in a state of dietary angst. By keeping your hunger (and internal chemicals) in check, you'll avoid the impetuous behaviours that send fat on an express ride to your belly.

YOU Will Make Mistakes

Look, we don't care how motivated you are, how willing you are, how inspired you are by Eva Longoria's body. Someday, and someday soon, a football-size muffin is going to get the better of you and nudge, bribe or cajole its way into your stomach. That's okay. Hear that? That's *okay.* You have to get past the concept that diets have *side effects* – that is, unexpected negative consequences. Instead, realize that eating plans have *effects* – offshoot actions, behaviours and emotions that are simply part of everyday living. One of those effects is that you will occasionally eat things that are nutritional cigarettes; while one may not hurt you, it can get you addicted to some bad behaviours. Because of that, waist management is about developing contingency plans – plans that allow you to make mistakes and then get back on the right road.

YOU Will Be Flexible – and Have Fun

Most of us want our diets to be a little like having the remote control: we want the power to make lots of choices, depending on everything from our mood to the time of day. It's clear from research that the most successful eating plans are low-maintenance: You can follow them with your family, and you won't feel overwhelmed by cravings. If you can do that, you'll get results. But try to stay on a diet where you feel isolated, then chances are that the result will feel like a miserable failure.

So now that we're about to begin, you're probably asking: what are we going to do, and how are we going to do it? Well, we're going to give you everything you need to make a body change – through a series of elegant and effective changes based on hard science – that will stick with you for your life. Simply, this book will serve as your lifelong waist-management, body-changing plan.

Best of all, when you put it all together and integrate automatic actions into your life, you'll live by the principles you need to stay fit and healthy, so that you can achieve and maintain exactly what you're striving for:

Your ideal body.

Chapter 1

THE IDEAL BODY

What your body is supposed to look like

Diet Myths

- Your body doesn't need any fat.
- Fast food is responsible for most of our fat problems.
- Dieting has to be hard.

The most common question heard among overweight people isn't 'Can I have more chips?' It's 'Why can't I lose weight?' While you may think you know the answer (severe pancake addiction), the real reason is biological:

We're actually hardwired to store some fat.

Our bodies have more systems that allow us to gain weight than to lose it. Historically, that served us well. Our ancestors gained and stored weight to survive periodic famines. Today, though, we've poisoned the systems that help us lose weight and empowered the ones that allow us to gain it – botching up our anatomy and turning our bodies into fat-storing machines. One of your goals will be to reprogram your body so that your internal systems can work the way they did when the greatest enemy we faced was a charging wildebeest, not a jumbo sausage roll.

The bodies of early man and woman looked like stereo-typical superheroes: strong, lean, muscular, able to jump snorting mammals in a single bound. In early times, our diets consisted of fruits, nuts, vegetables, tubers and wild meat – foods that were, for the most part, low in calories. The meat provided the protein, vitamins, minerals and fatty acids that helped them grow taller and develop larger brains, while the other foods gave them nutrients such as glucose, a simple sugar found in fruit and the complex carbohydrates of plants, that they needed to grow and develop, and for energy to move. And, of course, food was always fresh.

That's not to say our ancestors didn't enjoy their foods. They consumed their sugars through fruit, and they even splurged when they came across the Palaeolithic Cinnabon – a honeycomb. The difference between their splurges and ours? They came across the sweet treats only rarely; it's not as if they popped in for a 900-calorie sugar bomb every time they went shopping for a new buffalo hide. Add that to the fact that their definition of 'searching for food' included walking, stalking and chasing. It was a lot of work to get food, so they naturally burned many of the calories they consumed through the physical activity of hunting and gathering.

Another difference was that the meat our ancestors ate wasn't like the meat we know today. Theirs was low in fat and high in protein; ours often comes in the form of corn-fed cows pumped up to make fattier, tastier cuts. Truly wild

FACTOID

The difference between obese people and thin people isn't the number of fat cells but the size of these cells. You don't make more fat cells the fatter you get; you have the same number of fat cells you had as an adolescent. The only difference is that the fat globules within each cell increase as you store more fat. By the way, muscles work the same way: you don't make more muscle cells; the muscle cells get larger.

game has about 4 per cent fat, while now most commercially available beef has nine times that amount. (The theory behind protein-heavy diets like Atkins is that protein reduces overall food intake and could reduce calories as well. The flaw is that eating proteins dripping in saturated fat, like bacon, isn't exactly the same as eating the leaner, healthier forms of protein like chicken and fish.)

The result: our tribal forefathers and foremothers could eat anytime they could harvest or catch something, and still not put on excess weight.

The lesson: our ancestors never thought about a diet in the way we do – and their bodies had the approximate density of granite. Us? We obsess about diet more than red-carpet reporters obsess about designer dresses, and our bodies have the consistency of yogurt.

Still, we can't blame the advent of fast food for all of our weight issues. The downfall started in the pre-GA (pre-Golden Arches) era – over 10,000 years or so ago, when agriculture first appeared. Agriculture allowed us to make more advances than a 17-year-old boy in a cinema, but we paid a price for them. Besides sparing the lives of countless mammoths, the rise of agriculture ensured that we'd always have a steady supply of food – an advantage during times of famine, a disadvantage at the all-you-can-eat buffet. With a constant source of food, people became less nomadic, and communities grew closer together. While the average life span increased (thanks to the elimination of the extreme sport of tiger chasing, with, perhaps, some help from sanitation and immunization), agriculture also brought its share of downsides: more bacterial infections, shorter stature and rotting teeth that comes from eating refined sugar and less nutritious farm-raised food (overused soil depletes food of its nutrients). Our ancestors' diets shifted from vegetables and meat to grains from the farms, essentially hindering them from getting the diverse mix of protein and micronutrients needed for brain development.

The advent of agriculture essentially started the socio-logical shift that altered the way we lived – and the way we eat – up until this day. We could now produce food, so we could now produce what we wanted, not necessarily what we needed. Instead of making foods that could both complement our bodies and appeal to our taste buds, we started making ones that were kinder to our tongues and wallets than they were to our waists.

We're not in the business of trying to make you live like cavemen. What we should acknowledge, though, is that we

The Heavyweight Fight: Genetics versus Environment

It's easy to argue that lifestyle choices and lack of willpower are responsible for weight problems (it's the argument that lean people tend to make). But it doesn't explain the 95 per cent failure rate after two years of people who have lost 50 pounds or more; they had plenty of willpower to lose but regained the weight nonetheless.

Researchers argue that obesity is more genetically linked than any other trait except height – and at least 50 per cent of obesity cases clearly have genetic components. Our take: the waist control game requires two players – environment and genetics. Even if your genes have made you predestined for a life of taking up two seats, that doesn't mean you should abdicate control over your body. When you make the right behavioural and biological changes that we outline, you'll be able to stay healthy and avoid the bad side effects of excess weight, like diabetes, high blood pressure (hypertension) and arterial inflammation.

If you need to worry about losing two, three or even four stone, your problem is not likely to be genetic. Only when your excess weight exceeds seven stone would most doctors consider testing for genetic abnormalities. As the fight against obesity continues, we'll see more and more drug companies target genetic reasons for weight gain. That said, the onus still falls on you to improve your environment and your behaviours so that your genetics can work for you, not against you.

live in a world with free will and with temptations. Biologically, our bodies want us to eat right. But in today's society, our biological drive to be the right weight and to eat right can be overcome by stress or temptation (cavemen didn't have bad bosses or deadlines for annual reports).

And that has shifted many dietary decisions from biological necessities to psychological reactions. What we're going to do is teach you how to reprogram your body to work the way it's supposed to work – so that you eat to satisfy and to fuel rather than to console or excite. Controlling your fat isn't about being banished with a life sentence of broccoli florets. It's about teaching your body a little bit about the way our ancestors ate. Naturally and automatically.

YOU Tips!

Automate Your Eating

If your waist-management plan is going to work – as in really work, for your whole life – then eating right has to become as automatic as it was for our ancestors. That's not as insurmountable as it seems. Just look at one study from the *Journal of the American Medical Association*. Two groups were assigned two different diets. One went on a diet rich with good-for-you foods like wholegrains, fruits, vegetables, nuts and olive oil, foods found in the typical Mediterranean diet. The other group was not given any specific direction in terms of foods to eat but was instructed to consume specific percentages of fat, carbohydrates and protein daily. In short, they had to think a lot about preparing foods and dividing amounts, while the first group only had general guidelines about foods to eat.

The groups weren't given guidelines about how much to eat; they let their hunger levels dictate their hunger patterns. And when they did that, what happened? Without trying, the first group ate fewer calories, lost inches and dropped pounds.

YOU-reka!

The point: the people in the good-foods group ate the foods that naturally kept them satiated so their bodies could seek their playing weights (these are the foods we recommend in the YOU Diet). They didn't obsess about calories, and enabled their bodies to do what they're supposed to do: regulate the chemicals responsible for hunger and for satiety (more on this in Chapter 2).

Don't Undereat

When our ancestors couldn't find food and went for long periods of time without it, their bodies acted like a life preserver, storing fat in anticipation of the inevitable periods of famine. The same system works today.

YOU-reka!

When you try to 'diet' by going for long periods of time without eating or by eating far too few calories, your brain senses the starvation and sends an SOS signal through your body to store fat because famine is on its way. That's why people who go on extreme fasts and extremely low-calorie diets don't lose the expected weight. They store fat as a natural protective mechanism. To lose weight, you have to keep your body from switching into starvation mode. The only way to do it: eat often, in the form of frequent, healthy meals and snacks.

Plan Your Meals

Start every day knowing when and what you're going to eat. That way, you'll avert the 180-degree shift between starving and gorging that occurs when you skip meals. Our 14-day diet (in Chapter 12) will show you how to plan your meals so that you feed your body regularly to avoid extreme periods of overeating and undereating that can lead to a gain in weight and inches.

YOU Test: Remember Your Ancestry

Some people say their family has big bones or big cells. Some say their family has big appetites. Some say their family just has big fridges. If you gained weight as an adult, you can get a relatively accurate picture of what your ideal size should be by thinking about what you looked like when you were 18 (for women) or 21 (for men); a time when you were at your metabolically most efficient and when you weren't stapled to an office chair for 60 hours a week. Most people gain their weight between the ages of 21 and 60, so by looking at your size at 18 or 21, you'll have a good, though not quite scientific, idea of your factory settings. It's not perfect, but it's a thumbnail sketch of where you want to be. You can record your waist size (or closest guess) from when you were 18, but, more important, think about your shape. Ask your parents about their body sizes – or find pictures of them – when they were 18, to help give you a good idea of what you're supposed to look like.

YOU Test: Stand in Front of the Mirror, Naked, without Sucking in Your Belly

For some of you, this assignment may feel natural, but for most, the exercise is as uncomfortable as an economy-class airline seat. We're having you do this not to benefit the local Peeping Toms, but for two other reasons. First, we want you to realize that we're emphasizing healthy weight. Not fashion-magazine weight, not featherweight, but *healthy* weight. And we think that means you have to start getting comfortable with the fact that every woman isn't as light as a kite, and every man won't have the body of Matthew McConaughey. Where you want to be may not be *exactly* where your body wants you to be. We're not saying you need to accept a belly that looks like four gallons of melted ice cream, but we want you to get closer to your ideal health – and that means physically and emotionally.

Second, we want you to look at your body. Now draw an outline of your body shape (both from the side and front views). Ask a partner or close friend to look at the shape you drew and tell you – honestly – if that's approximately what your body looks like. (Your clothes can be back on at this point.) This is just a quality-control check to make sure you have an accurate self body image. (Those with eating disorders have very distorted body images, making it an obstacle for getting back to a healthy weight.) This might be the first time you've ever had to articulate things about what your body looks like – and that's good.

PART II

THE BIOLOGY OF FAT

Food, from start to finish – why our bodies want it, how we store it and how we burn it

Chapter 2

CAN'T GET NO SATISFACTION

The science of appetite

Diet Myths

- Hunger is primarily dictated by what's happening in your stomach.
- The biggest battle in dieting involves willpower.
- As long as a food is low-fat, it's not going to make you fat.

As much as an iPod bud in the ear, fat has become a normal part of our landscape. We see it *everywhere*. We see it tethered to a hunk of prime rib. We see it masquerading as peanut butter. We see it crammed into evening gowns or cascading over belt buckles. We've seen paparazzi-haunted celebrities gain it and lose it, lose it and gain it. And, if we can bear a confidence-crushing six seconds of nudity in front of a mirror, most of us have seen our own share of flesh that droops, sags or jiggles. So, reason would tell you that we should know as much about fat as we know about Angelina Jolie's private life. But we don't.

Of course, we know what it looks like, what it feels like and that it can be as bad for our health as a steak knife lodged in our hand. But few of us really know how fat works biologically – how a wonderfully yellow spongy cake morphs into the flab that conjoins our inner thighs, or how our skinny-as-a-straw friend can wolf down a meat-lover's supreme while we feel bloated if we as much as sniff four carrots.

Starting in this chapter and continuing throughout the rest of Part II, we'll show you the way that food travels – from the time your body wants you to eat it to the time it exercises squatter's rights on your hips. The best place to start? With your appetite. Appetite really comes in two forms: physiological signals that make you hungry and emotional coaxes that lure you to food.

In this chapter, we'll explore those physiological signals, because understanding and controlling your hunger and satiety signals will help you adopt a healthy eating plan. (We'll explore the psychological and emotional aspects in Part III.) Once you know that those mechanisms have much more powerful control over how you eat than do your taste buds, then you can make the behavioural, attitudinal and biological adjustments you need to live at your healthy weight.

Above all, there's one sign that will clue you in to whether you've become an effective processor of food.

That sign? Satisfaction.

As you change from *always* thinking about diet to *never* thinking about it, you will be reprogramming your body so that it's not your eyes, tongue or overzealous utensils that will guide you.

YOU-reka!

Instead, it will be the chemicals in your brain and body. By tuning in to your body's signals, you'll allow your anatomy to work the way it's supposed to: so that you'll never be famished, you'll never pop a button at the table and you'll never bounce between hunger extremes. Instead, you'll get a little hungry, you'll eat, you'll stop. Satisfied.

The Anatomy of Appetite

You'd think that the first place we'd start to talk about how appetite influences fat would be the spot that's covered by an XXXXL shirt. But to understand appetite, you have to navigate further north – to the place that may hold the least fat. In your brain, you'll find the hypothalamus, a key command centre for your body. Among the biological functions it controls are your temperature, your metabolism and your sex drive. Located in the centre of your brain, the hypothalamus (see Figure 2.1) also coordinates your behaviours that involve appetite – not just for food but also for thirst and even for sex. So while it may appear that call-to-duty signals come from your stomach growling or your loins tingling like a static shock, it's actually your brain that's sending out the signals that you crave either a quiche or a quickie. (At least one person we know helped curb an eating problem by having regular, monogamous, healthy

Fat's Bad Rap

Nobody likes body fat, especially when it beats you through the door by five or six seconds. But despite potentially serious consequences, fat, by nature, is good. (That's not a typo.) Besides helping Santa hopefuls land December jobs, it also helps your cells function and provides insulation. Most of your fat is stored in a reservoir throughout your body. You have drums and drums of it, sitting passively, just waiting to be burned. But you have another kind of fat, too. It's called brown fat and is usually found on the back of your neck and around your arteries (and has absolutely nothing to do with how much chocolate you eat). This increases in outdoor workers during cold spells to protect them from the weather; it insulates our vital organs. Though you have a fairly small percentage of brown fat as an adult, about one-third of fat in babies is brown fat, and it's used primarily to keep them warm. What makes brown fat different?

Brown fat is *alive*. It has nerve fibres, like any organ, and it also has leptin receptors. When the level of this hormone goes up, it turns on energy consumption in the brown fat and burns it. This is important because it shows that the right leptin levels can signal you to immediately get rid of this fat. And it's also symbolic of the inherent goodness of body fat – when it's found in the right amounts.

sex. When the appetite function for sex was satisfied, the appetite function for food was diverted.)

Hidden in your hypothalamus, you have a satiety centre that regulates your appetite. It is controlled by two counterbalancing chemicals that are located side by side.

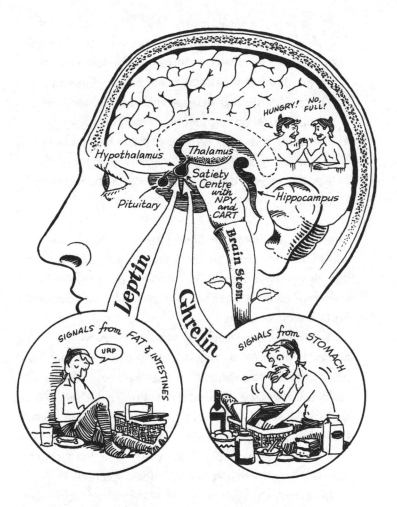

Figure 2.1 Food Fight

In your hypothalamus, you have hunger and satiety chemicals. The hormone leptin goes to the satiety centre to make you feel full and satisfied, while the signal from the hormone ghrelin makes you want to eat, gorge and slobber over your every feast.

- The satiety chemicals led by CART (the C stands for cocaine and the A for amphetamine, since these drugs put this chemical into overdrive). CART stimulates the surrounding hypothalamus to increase metabolism, reduce appetite and increase insulin to deliver energy to muscle cells rather than be stored as fat.
- The eating chemicals driven by NPY (a protein called neuropeptide Y). NPY has the opposite effect on the hypothalamus; it decreases metabolism and increases appetite.

Think of these two command chemicals as any game or sport that involves attack and defence, like football, draughts or even dating. The attackers are always trying to make advances and score points, while the defenders protect their territory.

Your eating chemicals play in attack. They want as many points as possible, so they fire off those signals for your body to score: eat, eat, eat, calories, calories, calories. The biological message: prevent starvation by eating. Meanwhile, your satiety chemicals play in defence, like a goalkeeper or a protective parent. They send the messages to your brain that you're full, to shield you from steadily pumping bacon-wrapped scallops down your gullet.

In a perfect system, your attackers and defenders complement each other; you get the foods you need and stop when you've had enough. Unfortunately for everyone except elastic-waistband manufacturers, a lot of things can mess up those systems (many of which we'll discuss in a moment). But these obstacles aren't insurmountable. You

FACTOID

As you get older, you have fewer leptin receptors in your hypothalamus – meaning that you have fewer satiety signals, which makes you more prone to gaining weight.

can take comfort (and find motivation) in the fact that your body wants you to reach your goals. Your body doesn't want to be bigger than it should be. Your body doesn't want lots of excess fat. Take the case of rats made obese by force-feeding. When they're allowed to eat freely, they go back to their control weight. *They eat what they should eat, without thinking.* Same goes for starving rats. When allowed to eat again, they don't gorge. They naturally go back to their control weight. And we know from years and years of research that what rats do is a pretty fair indication of what humans will do under the same circumstances. (Humans, of course, will do what rats do when they're motivated only by biology. A rat isn't upset by stress at home or work, which is why controlling the emotional aspect of eating plays such a big role in effective waist management, as we'll discuss in Part III.)

YOU-reka!
If you can allow your body and brain to subconsciously do the work of controlling your eating, you'll naturally gravitate towards your ideal playing weight. You do it by developing a well-trained defence that naturally balances the attack. When you do, you'll win the diet game every time, whether you have willpower or not.

The Hunger On and Off Switches

Duct tape over your mouth isn't how your body regulates food intake. Your body does it naturally through the communication of substances controlled by your brain. Although there are many hunger- and obesity-related hormones waiting to be discovered, there's enough evidence to suggest that two hormones have as much influence for dictating our hunger and satiety levels as a head coach does on attackers and defenders.

Lovin' Leptin: the Hormone of Satisfaction

Fat produces a chemical signal in your blood that tells you to stop eating. Left to its own devices, fat is self-regulating; the problem occurs when we override our internal monitoring system and continue to stuff ourselves long after we're no longer hungry. Your body knows when it's had enough, and it prevents you from wanting any more food on top of that. How does fat curb appetite? Through one of the most important chemicals in the weight-reduction process: leptin, a protein secreted by stored fat. In fact, if leptin is working the way it should, it gives you a double whammy in the fight against fat. The stimulation of leptin (the word comes from the Greek word for 'thin') shuts off your hunger *and* stimulates you to burn more calories – by stimulating CART.

But our bodies aren't always perfect, and leptin doesn't always work the way it's supposed to. In some research, when leptin was given to mice, their appetites decreased, as expected. When it was given to people, they initially got thin, but then something strange happened: They overcame the surge of leptin and stopped losing weight. This indicates that our bodies have the ability to override leptin's message that our tank is full. How? When leptin tells your defence – the satiety chemicals – to kick in and

---

FACTOID

Neuropeptide Y is a stress hormone that increases with severe or prolonged stress. This may be why some people in chronically stressful situations tend to gain weight. Testosterone, the male sex hormone, seems to stimulate NPY secretion, while the female sex hormone, oestrogen, seems to have a varying effect depending on the stage of a woman's cycle.

protect you against stray bonbons, the pleasure centre in your brain says, 'Uh, yeah, three more this-a-way.' That surge from the pleasure centre, which we'll discuss in more detail in Part III, can overrule leptin's messages that you're full. That's called leptin resistance (there's another form of leptin resistance as well, which happens when cells stop accepting leptin's messages). Most obese people, by the way, have high leptin levels; it's just that their bodies have the second form of leptin resistance – they don't receive and respond to leptin signals.

That doesn't mean leptin is always on the losing end of this chemical battle.

YOU-reka!

The challenge is to let leptin do its job so that the brain demands less food. One way to do it: walk for 30 minutes a day and build a little muscle (that's part of our activity plan in Part IV). When you lose some weight, your cells become more sensitive and responsive to leptin.

Ghrelin is the Gremlin: the Hormone of Hunger

Your stomach and intestines do more than hold food and produce Richter-worthy belches. When your stomach's empty, they release a feisty little chemical called ghrelin. When your stomach's growling, it's this gremlin of a hormone that's controlling your body's attackers; it sends desperate messages that you need more points. Ghrelin makes you want to eat – by stimulating NPY.

YOU-reka!

To make things worse, when you diet through deprivation, the increased ghrelin secretion sends even more signals to eat, overriding your willpower and causing chemical reactions that give you little choice but to line your tongue with bits of pork pie.

Ghrelin also promotes eating by increasing the secretion of growth hormone (*ghre* is the Indo-European root word for 'growth'). So when you increase ghrelin levels, you stimulate that growth hormone to kick in, and growth hormone builds you not only up but out as well.

Your stomach secretes ghrelin in pulses every half hour, sending subtle chemical impulses to your brain – almost like subliminal biological messages (carrot cake, carrot cake, carrot cake). When you're really hungry or dieting, those messages come fast – every 20 minutes or so – and they're also amplified. So you get more signals and stronger signals that your body wants food. After long periods, your body can't ignore those messages. That's why chocolate biscuits usually trump willpower, and that's why deprivation dieting can never work.

YOU-reka!

It's impossible to fight the biology of your body. The chemical vicious cycle stops when you eat; when your stomach fills is when you reduce your ghrelin levels, thus reducing your appetite. So if you think your job is to resist biology, you're going to lose that battle time after time. But if you can reprogram your body so that you keep those ghrelin gremlins from making too much noise, then you've got a chance to keep your tank feeling like it's always topped up.

Sometimes, it may seem like we don't have much control over the chemical reactions taking place within our arteries or inside our brains. But just as you can control things like cholesterol and blood pressure by changing the foods you eat or altering your behaviours, you can also control the satiety centre of your brain. How? Through your choice of foods.

At least as far as your body is concerned, foods are drugs; they're foreign substances that come in and switch around all those natural chemical processes going about their business. When your body receives foods, different chemical reactions take place, and messages get sent throughout your system – turning on some things, turning off others. While your body internally gives orders, you set the tone and direction of those orders through the food you're feeding it. Eat the right foods (like nuts), and your hormones will keep you feeling satisfied. But eat the wrong foods (like simple sugars), and you'll cause your body to go haywire hormonally, and that ends up with one result: the next notch in your belt.

A major gang leader against your body is fructose, found in high-fructose corn syrup (HFCS), a sweetener in many processed foods. Here's how it works: when you eat calories from healthy sources, they turn off your desire to eat by inhibiting production of NPY or by producing more CART. But fructose in HFCS, which sweetens our soft drinks and salad dressings, isn't seen by your brain as a normal food.

Because your brain doesn't see any of the fructose in the thousands of HFCS-containing foods as excess calories or as NPY suppressants, your body wants you to keep eating. Foods with fructose – which may in fact be labelled as low-fat – make you both hungry and unable to shut off your appetite. They are also rich sources of calories. So you constantly get the signal that you're hungry, even after you've jammed your gut with two baskets of calorie-laden, fructose-loaded biscuits.

YOU Tips!

Read the label

You should read food labels as attentively as you read the stock market or your horoscope. Don't eat foods that have any of the following listed as one of the first five ingredients:

Food Fight: the Ghrelin versus Leptin Grudge Match

So now let's get back to that attack and defence. The natural state is for you to have a give-and-take relationship between your eating and satiety chemicals – between your ghrelin and leptin levels – to influence NPY and CART, respectively. It's the relationship between the impulse that says, 'I'll take a large pepperoni with extra cheese,' and the one that says, 'No more passengers, this belly is full.'

This battle over eating isn't between your willpower and the Belgian waffles; it's between your brain chemicals. The NPY is the villain – encouraging you to buffets, driving you to the pantry, pointing its chemical finger to the convenience foods – while CART is your dietary guardian angel, which encourages a cascade of allies to keep you full and satisfied. Think of the two substances – NPY and CART – competing for the same parking space, the one that will ultimately determine whether or not you eat. They both arrive at the same time and want that space. Either more NPY or more CART sneaks into the spot, thus sending the all-important go or stop signal to your brain to influence the hormones that make you feel full or hungry.

Here's how they all work together: ghrelin works in the short term, sending out those hunger signals twice an hour. Leptin, on the other hand, works in the long term, so if you can get your leptin levels high, you'll have a greater ability to keep your hunger and appetite in check. Isn't that great? Leptin can outrank ghrelin – to keep you from feeling like feasting on anything short of fingernails every few minutes. If you focus on ways to influence your leptin levels, and, more importantly, leptin effects (through leptin sensitivity), your brain (through CART) will help control your hunger.

- Simple sugars
- Enriched, bleached or refined flour (this means it's stripped of its nutrients)
- HFCS (high-fructose corn syrup – a four-letter word).

Putting them into your body is like dunking your mobile phone in a glass of water. It'll cause your system to short out your hormones and send your body confusing messages about eating.

Choose Unsaturated over Saturated

Meals high in saturated fat (that's one of the aging fats) produce lower levels of leptin than low-fat meals with the exact same calories. That indicates you can increase your satiety and decrease hunger levels by avoiding saturated fats found in such sources as high-fat meats (like sausage), baked goods and whole-milk dairy products.

Don't Confuse Thirst with Hunger

The reason some people eat is because their satiety centres are begging for attention. But sometimes, those appetite centres want things to quench thirst, not to fill the stomach. Thirst could be caused by hormones in the gut, or it could be a chemical response to eating; eating food increases the thickness of your blood, and your body senses the need to dilute it. A great way to counteract your hormonal reaction to food is to make sure that your response to thirst activation doesn't contain unnecessary, empty calories – like the ones in soft drinks or alcohol. Your thirst centre doesn't care whether it's getting zero-calorie water or a mega-calorie frap.

YOU-reka!

When you feel hungry, drink a glass or two of water first, to see if that's really what your body wants.

Avoid the Alcohol Binge

For weight loss, avoid drinking excessive alcohol – not solely because of its own calories, but also because of the calories it inspires you to consume later. Alcohol lowers your inhibition, so you end up feeling like you can eat anything and everything you see. Limiting yourself to one alcoholic drink a day has a protective effect on your arteries but could still cost you pounds, since it inhibits leptin.

Watch Your Carbs

Eating a super-high-carb diet increases NPY, which makes you hungry, so you should ensure that less than 50 per cent of your diet comes from carbohydrates. Make sure that most of your carbs are complex, such as wholegrains and vegetables.

Stay – Va-va-voom – Satisfied

In any waist-management plan, you can stay satisfied. Not in the form of a dripping double cheeseburger but in the form of safe, healthy, monogamous sex. Sex and hunger are regulated through the brain chemical NPY. Some have observed that having healthy sex could help you control your food intake; by satisfying one appetite centre, you seem to satisfy the other.

Manage Your Hormonal Surges

There will be times when you can't always control your hormone levels; when ghrelin outslugs your leptin, and you feel hungrier than a lion on a bug-only diet. Develop a list of emergency foods to satisfy you when cravings get the better of you – things like V8 juice, a handful of nuts, pieces of fruit, cut-up vegetables or even a little guacamole.

Chapter 3

EATER'S DIGEST

How food travels through your body

Diet Myths

- Fat turns to fat, protein turns to muscle and carbs turn to energy.
- The fullness of your stomach is what tells you to stop eating.
- Sugar gives you an instant high to help combat hunger.

Once your brain tells you to eat, that's exactly what you do. You eat. Maybe you gorge. Maybe you nibble. And then maybe you forget about that hefty cheeseburger until it ends up on the back of your thighs. But in between mouth and thighs, there's an amazing system of digestion that takes place – a system that determines whether that food gets burned, stored or expelled faster than a delinquent school pupil.

Now that you know the biochemical reasons why you shuttle food to your mouth, it's time to start exploring the biology of what happens to food once it's in there. In this

chapter, we'll discuss what happens in the early p
your digestive system, and in the next chapter, w
discuss the effects of food as it interacts with the rest of
your digestive organs.

Your Digestive Motorway

On your gastrointestinal motorway, everything enters via
your physiological toll booth: your mouth. The nutritious
powerhouses slide through the express toll to give you the
power, energy, stamina and strength to live your life. Toxic
(though sometimes tasty) foods can enter too, but you'll
pay a heavier toll later for the damage they do along the
way and after. Throughout its journey, your food and all of
its nutrients (and toxins) will pull over at various organs,
slow down on winding roads, speed up, merge with other
nutrients and even get pulled over by the bowel brigade
for nutritional offences. (See Figure 3.1.)

During every trip, your food hits a symbolic three-
pronged fork in the road:

- Either it will be broken down and picked up by your
  bloodstream and liver to be used as energy.
- Or it will be broken down and stored as fat.
- Or it will be processed as waste and directed to nature's
  recycling pot: the porcelain junkyard.

art of
e'll

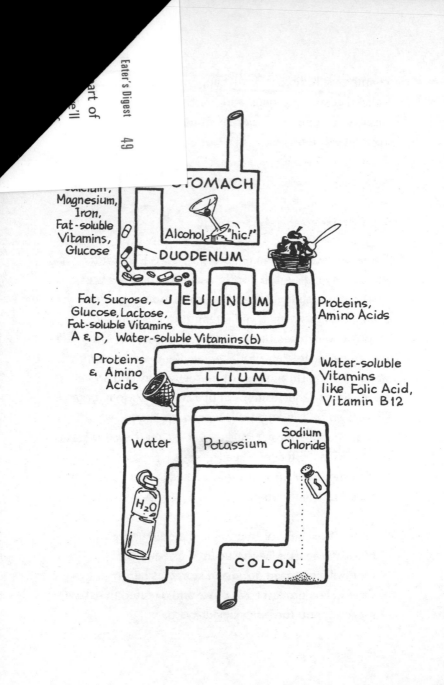

Figure 3.1 Gutting It Out

Food pulls over at various spots in the intestinal track, so disease of these areas can cause nutritional deficiencies even if two people are eating identical foods. Not all of the nutrients that come from food and supplements get absorbed in the same place; they're absorbed throughout your gastrointestinal tract:

Stomach: alcohol
Duodenum: (first part of the small intestine; takes off from the stomach) calcium, magnesium, iron, fat-soluble vitamins A and D, glucose
Jejunum: (middle part of the small intestine) fat, sucrose, lactose, glucose, proteins, amino acids, fat-soluble vitamins A and D, water-soluble vitamins like folic acid
Ileum: (last part of the small intestine; leads to large bowel) proteins, amino acids, water-soluble vitamins like folic acid, vitamin B12
Colon: (also known as the large bowel) water, potassium, sodium chloride

Here's how the system starts: before a morsel even reaches the tollbooth, your body has a radar gun to let you know that food is coming – powered by such physiological cues as sight, smell and the fact that you've been drooling like an overheated Saint Bernard at the thought of garlic bread smothered in mozzarella. In response to that sensory information, glands in your mouth start to secrete enzymes to help break down your food; then your stomach quickly starts pumping out stomach acid to help prepare your body for the digestion process.

Now, don't underestimate your stamp licker as a player in this digestion process. Back in the days of buffalo-hide cocktail dresses, people relied on their tongues (and their noses) for survival; if it tasted good, then it was safe, and if it tasted like dinosaur dung, then it could be poisonous or toxic.

We do the same things, but in slightly different ways. Since our bodies use our senses to process information, we rely on our tongue for information about food. The information we acquire sends messages to the brain, and then the brain sends messages to our forks: keep eating or stop eating. That message largely comes from our five tastes (sweet, sour, salty, bitter and unami, which recognizes the inherent deliciousness in foods like juicy filet mignon), but it also comes from what we smell. Some researchers say that three-quarters of how we 'taste' certain foods actually comes from how we smell it. What's this have to do with your waist growing? For one, there's the obvious: the more you like a bad-for-you food, the more likely you are to keep eating it. But the genetics of taste and taste buds may play an even more subtle and fascinating role. As you'll see on page 66 ('Are You a Supertaster?'), the physiological makeup of your tongue could make you more or less disposed to eating good or bad foods.

Unlike other animals, we waste very little energy eating because of our highly efficient, perfectly opposing molars. The powerful crushing motion helps us extract every possible calorie from our food. Other animals waste or burn a lot of calories while they eat because their teeth do not efficiently mush the food when they move prey to belly. In humans, once that food actually does breeze past

FACTOID

Eating nuts does not create the calorie intake that you might expect, because 5–15 per cent of the calories are not absorbed by the intestinal system. That's because the nuts' skin and how well we chew nuts influence digestion. An added bonus: the slow release of calories throughout the intestinal system leads to prolonged satiety.

the toll booth, it accelerates onto the on-ramp of the oesophagus – that's the tube that links your mouth to the motorway that is your gastrointestinal system.

After your Double Whopper slides down the on-ramp, it has to make a tricky merge in the form of a sharp turn to enter the stomach. That angle – the gastroesophageal junction – is what keeps stomach acid from spilling back into your oesophagus and making your chest feel like an arson victim. (When you have extra fat in your belly, that angle is prised open, allowing acid to spill upwards and cause heartburn.) Once your Whopper chunks have entered your stomach, serious digestion begins. The food is held in your stomach until your body directs it to the small intestine, where most of the nutrients are absorbed and passed along to the rest of your body through your bloodstream (to the liver, which is the next stop for absorbed nutrients), or to the large intestine on the way to evacuation.

Food Processor: How Your Body Breaks Down Nutrients

In terms of weight gain, a calorie is a calorie is a calorie. Calories not used immediately by your body for energy are either eliminated as waste or stored as fat. But that doesn't mean that all calories are treated equally by your body. For example, protein and fibre with high water content have a great effect on satiety, and simple carbohydrates have the least effect on satiety. (Fat, by the way, has an effect on satiety similar to that of protein and fibre, which is why low-fat diets leave people hungry all the

---

Oh, the Gall

Your gallbladder may seem as unnecessary as bad goatees, but one of its functions is to help store bile – that digestive juice that helps your body absorb nutrients. Obese people have a greater than 50 per cent chance of developing gallstones. Why? An overworked liver caused by being overweight makes bile, which is more like sludge than liquid, and predisposes them to developing stones. It's also more likely that you'll develop stones when you lose weight fast, like after weight-loss surgery – because the gallbladder doesn't empty enough when it doesn't see any fat. So it's not uncommon for a surgeon to remove the gallbladder during a gastric bypass procedure. The risk factors for developing the painful stones are easy to remember, because they sound like an R&B group. They're the four Fs: female, fertile, fat and forty. (We don't mean this to be a gender issue, but the fact is that women are more likely to have gallstone symptoms than men.)

time.) When it comes to converting calories, your body processes fat most efficiently – meaning that you actually keep more of it, because your body doesn't need to expend as many calories trying to store it. On the flip side, your body works hard to process protein, to make it highly flammable to your body's metabolic furnace.

Contrary to popular belief, not all ingested protein becomes muscle, and not all the fat in your food gets stored on your hips. Everything has the potential to turn into fat if it's not used by your body for energy at the exact time it is absorbed through your intestines. And energy is energy is energy. Here's how the different nutrients are processed:

Simple Sugars (as in a cola)

When sugar, which is quickly absorbed and sent to the liver, meets the liver in the digestion process, the liver tells your body to turn that sugar into a fat if it can't be used immediately for energy.

Complex Carbohydrates (as in wholegrain foods)

They take longer to digest, so there's a slower release of the carbohydrates that have been converted in your bowel to sugar to become sugar in your bloodstream. That means your digestive system is not stressed as much. Still, if your body can't use this slower sugar when it's released, it gets converted to fat.

Protein (as in meat)

It gets broken down into small amino acids, which then go to the liver. If the liver can't send them to your muscles (say, if you're not exercising and don't need them for muscle growth or maintenance), then, yes, they get converted to glucose, which then gets converted to fat if you can't use it for energy.

Fat (as in cheesecake)

It gets broken into smaller particles of fat and gets absorbed as fat. Good fats (like those found in nuts and fish) decrease your body's inflammatory response, and bad fats increase it. That inflammatory response, which we'll explain in the next chapter, is a contributing factor to obesity and its complications. If you're exercising and have used up all readily available carbohydrates (sugar), your muscles can use fat for energy, which is a great way to erode your love handles.

Your Digestive Motorway: the Main Drag

At the bottom of your stomach and top of your intestines, your food hits an important traffic signal: it's the red light that tells your brain you're full and don't need another large order of onion rings (or the cheese sauce for dipping or the beer to wash it down). That red light is delivered by the vagus nerve, which is a large nerve that comes from the brain and stimulates the contraction of the stomach (see Figure 3.2). The vagus nerve is also the main cable controlling the parasympathetic system, which is the relaxation section of your nervous system. The key messenger switching the vagus on is a peptide produced in your gastrointestinal tract called CCK, which is released when your bowel senses fat. Technically, it stands for cholecystokinin, but for our purposes, let's think of it as the Crucial Craving Killer because its main purpose is to tell your brain via the vagus nerve that your stomach feels fuller than a *Baywatch* bathing suit.

Without having to go through the chemical pathways of your body (your bloodstream), CCK acts as a very direct message and indicator of your fullness. (Remember, leptin is more of a long-term indicator of your satiety; CCK provides a very short-term, intense message.)

After the food spends some time in your stomach, it will slowly leave that reservoir and go into the small intestine via the duodenum, the first part of your intestines that comes right after the stomach. That's when CCK puts up a digestive detour sign, in a very clear physical signal that makes you feel full. It causes the pylorus – the opening at the end of the stomach – to slam shut; that keeps food from moving into the small bowel. That's how your stomach gets full physically and how you feel full mentally. One interesting note: high-saturated-fat diets lead to less CCK sensitivity, so you do not feel as full as you should after eating a steak.

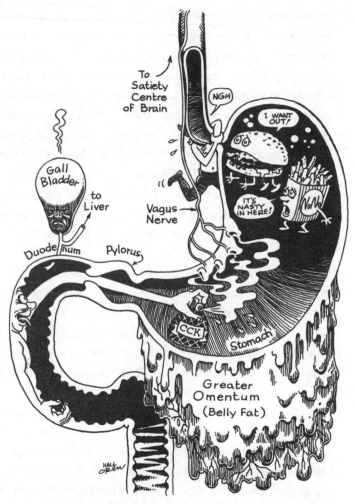

Figure 3.2 Stop Sign

Food entering the small bowel stimulates release of the substance CCK into the wall of the stomach. That's where the vagus nerve senses that we're full and informs the satiety centre in our brains to tell our hand to put down the buttered popcorn.

After the stomach, your food enters the small intestine and has a head-on collision with bile. Bile is the thick green digestive fluid that's secreted by the liver, stored in the gallbladder and released into the small intestine. (CCK also has a third effect: it's what causes the gallbladder to contract.) After fat is broken down into smaller particles by substances called lipases, which are released by the pancreas, these tiny particles interact with bile to form a compound that is easily absorbed by the cells of your body. Bile surrounds the fat in our meal like soap surrounds grease on our hands so it can be scrubbed from the intestinal wall and better digested and absorbed.

Once it reaches the bloodstream, food continues to influence how hungry you may feel. Elevated blood sugar sends your brain the message that it's time to take your plate to the sink and hit the sofa. When your blood sugar is low, that's what stimulates hunger.

Many of us get into trouble when we eat foods with simple sugars (think soft drinks, jelly, cake). Simple sugars create a rebounding effect. You feel lethargic so you eat a Mars Bar. The sugar surge works like an electrical jolt, and you instantly feel more energetic. But less than two hours later, that energy surge (in the form of elevated blood sugar levels) plummets, and then you feel lethargic again. Your conclusion? You must need another Mars Bar. That rebound effect (combined with the desire for the taste that's stimulated by the pleasure centre in your brain) can put your body in biological turmoil, where you eat to feel better, though what you're eating is actually making you feel sluggish, so you swirl and swirl around, always feeling like you need to eat.

YOU-reka!

At the bottom end of your small intestine (before it joins your large intestine), food hits the ileal brake – another signal that you're full. At this juncture there's a traffic signal that slows the passage of the slurry of intestinal contents from the small intestine to the large intestine. It's called the ileocaecal valve. The squeezing required to overcome this traffic signal valve is reduced naturally by some foods, since your body feels that you're still digesting and not ready to evacuate those foods yet. Very little absorption of nutrients occurs in the colon, so once the food passes the ileocaecal valve, not much more happens except that you reabsorb water while consolidating the waste you've formed. The result: you have a traffic jam in your gut, and if you try to send more cars down the road, the problem's only going to turn into a fuller feeling. It's one of the reasons why fibre kills cravings, because fibre slows down the transit of food from your small intestine to your large intestine, keeping that full feeling. In the next chapter, we'll pick up the rest of the digestive journey in the intestines, where some of the key fat-storing processes take place.

The System of Satisfaction

Though it may seem that we have endless reasons to eat –
to celebrate holidays, to beat stress, to pass the time –
there's only one real reason why we need food: for energy.
That energy allows our organs to function, our muscles to
move and our bodies to keep warm. And to a large extent,
our brains help control how we convert food to energy. To
help understand the process that your body goes through
to use energy, we'll break down the metabolic path into
two phases.

Digestive Phase

Your hypothalamus orchestrates this phase of metabolism
by receiving signals from throughout your body about
whether you're hungry or not, so that your body can use
energy to power itself. Here's how: your body has a short-
term reservoir for energy in the form of glycogen, a carbohydrate primarily stored in your liver and muscles. After
eating, when you have glucose (sugar) and insulin (the
hormone produced in the pancreas to transport glucose),
your body uses all of the glucose it needs for immediate
fuel but takes the rest and stores it as glycogen. If your
blood glucose level falls, your pancreas stops releasing
insulin – and then releases another G substance,
glucagon, which converts the stored energy (glycogen) to
sugar (glucose). So the effect is that when your intestinal
fuel tank empties of sugar (in other words, when our

ancestors were fasting between bison hunts), your body is still able to supply crucial energy to your central nervous system by converting glycogen to glucose.

Fasting Phase

When you're sleeping or go for long periods without eating, your body needs to have a supply of energy to keep your organs functioning. Once you use up all of your available glucose during the digestive phase of metabolism (your body stores only about 300 calories in the short-term glycogen reservoir), it taps a long-term reservoir: fatty tissue in the form of triglycerides (molecules that include a carbohydrate-containing glycerol). This keeps you going until you break the fast with breakfast.

YOU Tips!

Slow the Process

If you have a little of the right kinds of fat just before you eat, you can trick your hormonal system by sending the signal to your brain that you're full. If you eat a little fat 20 minutes before your meal (70 calories or so of fat in the form of six walnuts, 12 almonds or 20 peanuts), you'll stimulate production of CCK, which will both communicate with your brain and slow your stomach from emptying to keep you feeling full. (CCK release and ghrelin reduction take about 20 minutes to kick in and take about 65 calories of fat to stimulate.) That way, you'll be able to sit down for a meal and eat for pleasure, not for hunger – which is one way to ensure you'll eat less. The average person is finished eating well before their satiety signals kick in, thus counteracting any possibility that their hormones can help them. For the same reason, you should eat slowly. If you down your food faster than a vacuum cleaner, you won't allow your satiety hormones time to kick in.

Set the Early Fibre Alarm

Many of us may associate fibre with better health and increased toilet time, but fibre is the speed bump of your gastrointestinal motorway. It slows everything right down. Technically, it works by slowing the transit of food across the ileocaecal valve, keeping your stomach fuller for longer. The result: a greater feeling of satiety and an increase of appetite-suppressing CCK-like signals. While you should aim for around 30 grams of fibre a day, the key is bulking up in the morning. Studies show that consuming fibre in the morning (at breakfast) makes you less hungry in late afternoon – a notorious sweet-sucking, diet-busting time of day. Great sources of breakfast fibre include oatmeal, cereal, wholegrains and fruit. (You'll note that every breakfast in the YOU Diet – see Part IV – has a lot of fibre in it, whether it's the cereal or the vegetables in an egg white omelette or the wholewheat bread. And morning snacks, like an apple, also have fibre.)

Besides controlling blood sugar levels and decreasing insulin levels, fibre also reduces calorie intake for up to 18 hours a day. Start with 1–2 grams of dietary fibre before meals and at bedtime and slowly increase to 5 grams. (If you add it all at once, you'll produce more gas than a Saudi oil field.) The supplement konjac root also seems to have a fibre-related effect. One study showed a nearly six-pound weight loss in eight weeks for those who ate 1 gram of it an hour before their meals.

Step Down to the Plate

Monstrous portion sizes are one of our stomach's biggest enemies: Studies show that when you're served bad foods in large containers, you'll eat up to one-third more than if you were served in smaller containers. By getting served in larger popcorn boxes, bigger dishes and taller cups, we've automatically been tricked into thinking that availability should dictate how much we eat, rather than physical hunger. You don't have to go through drastic changes to make small ones. Start by changing your serving plates to the nine-inch variety to give yourself the visual and psychological clue that you're full when your physical appetite has been sated. That's important, because studies show visual clues help determine how full you are, in that you may not feel satisfied until your plate is clean, no matter how large the plate is. That's also reason never to eat directly out of a box or carton and always to remember that one serving size of a food is often about the size of a fist.

Slow Down

Stomach growling stimulates appetite, but growling does-n't really tell you how hungry you are. It tells you to eat, but not how much to eat. That's why meal size is so important. You're hardwired to eat, but you're not hardwired to eat a lot. Having a big meal quickly won't stop you from wanting to eat a few hours later. So slow down and let your CCK act; it takes about 20 minutes after the nuts to decrease your desire to eat.

Add Pepper

Red pepper, when eaten early in the day, decreases food intake later in the day. Some credit the ingredient capsaicin for being the catalyst for decreasing overall calorie intake and for increasing metabolism. It also appears to work by inhibiting sensory information from the intestines from reaching the brain, which is particularly effective in reducing appetite in low-fat diets. Capsaicin works by killing – or at least stunning – the messages that you're hungry. So add red peppers to your egg-white omelette.

YOU Test: Are You a Supertaster?

We all know that foods we like may send others seeking gas masks. But your tongue-related genetics may play an even bigger role in waist management.

If you're classified as a 'supertaster', you tend not to eat fruits and vegetables because they may taste very bitter, thereby putting yourself at a higher risk of certain diseases and colon polyps because you're not getting the nutrients from fruits and vegetables. You should supplement your diet with a multivitamin to ensure you're getting the right nutrients, as well as use fruits and veggies to enliven other things – as in salads and desserts and as moisturizers on breads (tomato ketchup works great here). And if you're an 'undertaster', you may be more prone to eating (and overeating) sweets because it takes more of a taste to satiate you. By the way, researchers say about 25 per cent of us are supertasters and 25 per cent are undertasters, while the rest of us are normal tasters.

Which taster are you?

The Saccharin Test

Mix one pack of saccharin into two-thirds of a cup of water; that's about the size of a tennis ball. Now taste the water. You'll probably taste a mix of both bitter and sweet, but see which taste is stronger. If sweet is dominant, then it means you're probably an undertaster, and if bitter is dominant, it means you're probably a supertaster. If it's a tie, you are like half the population. To be sure, you may have to do the test more than once to tease out differences.

The Blue Tongue Test

Wipe a swab of blue food dye on your tongue and see the small circles of pink-coloured tissue that polka-dot the newly painted blue canvas. Those are your papillae. Then put a piece of paper – with a 4-millimetre hole – over your tongue. Using a magnifying glass, count the little pink dots you see in the hole. If you have fewer then five dots, it means you're an undertaster, while more than 30 indicate you're probably a supertaster.

Chapter 4

GUT CHECK

The dangerous battles of inflammation in your belly

Diet Myths

- Your stomach is the place where you store your belly fat.
- Diets are mostly about calorie control.
- Your brain is the only part of your body that reacts emotionally to food.

We all know about the daily skirmishes that play out in the battle against obesity. You versus the salad dressing, you versus the dessert trolley and, in the title fight, your bum versus your jeans. But it would be a mistake to think that every weight-loss war happens at the table or in the privacy of your own wardrobe. In fact, millions of little firefights break out inside your gut every time you eat or drink – and these are the most influential battles in your personal crusade against excess weight. Deep inside your éclair-encrusted gut, you have cells and chemicals that react and respond to food in two ways: as an ally or as an enemy.

As we move along in our digestive journey to the second half of our digestive system, we'll explore these battles and how they influence your waistline. When interrogating nutrients as they pass through your digestive system, your body classifies them by what kind of inflammatory effect they have; the enemies contribute to inflammation, and the allies help to reduce it.

We're not just talking about the inflammation that happens when your belly balloons to the size of a conference centre, or the inflammation that happens to your joints if you have arthritis. We're talking about the chemical reaction of inflammation that happens within your bloodstream and is an underlying cause of weight gain. This process is like the rusting of our bodies. Just like metal rusts when exposed to oxygen, inflammation is caused when oxygen free radicals (no political affiliation) attack innocent bystanders in our bodies.

Inflammation happens on many different levels and through several different mechanisms, many of them to do with food. Not only can you get inflammation through allergies to food, but you can also get inflammation in the rest of your body – through the way your liver responds to saturated and trans fats, and through the way your body and belly fat respond to such toxins as cigarettes and stress. In turn, these inflammatory responses can cause things like hypertension, high cholesterol and insulin resistance – and *those* inflammatory responses influence

How Tolerant Are You?

With more than 100 million neurons in your intestines, gastrointestinal pain is immediate, but the level of discomfort you feel depends on your genetics; specifically on your tolerance of or allergies to certain foods and your genetic disposition for feeling the effects of those land mines. While there are certainly pharmaceutical solutions for dealing with the digestive explosions, there are also foods that produce an anti-inflammatory effect and can come in and put out the fire (see YOU Tips). During these inflammatory firefights, your intestines are contracting too much, or are being dilated – a painful process that works through the vagus nerve. Too much stimulation or distension of the bowel is what causes the pain. Some of us are less sensitive to those internal motions, so we may not always be getting the clue from our gut. These are some of the more common GI firestorms involving food intolerance:

■ **Enzyme deficiencies:** When your intestines lack enzymes to metabolize specific foods like milk, grains or beans, the food remains undigested, so you start feeding your intestines' ravenous bacteria. The result: lots of intestinal dilation and wind. The most common of these is lactose intolerance (the lack of gastrointestinal agreement with dairy products), and a close second is an allergy to the protein gluten from wheat (and rye and barley; nutritional good guys). As an example, when you lack the enzyme lactase, the sugar lactose in the

the total-body mother of all inflammation in your arteries, which leads to heart disease. (We'll discuss these at length in the next chapter.)

milk reaching your intestine is not metabolized, so it's presented to your intestinal bacteria, which metabolize the lactose in your intestines, producing a lot of wind.

■ **General gastrointestinal disorders:** Problems like irritable bowel syndrome, which causes gut-related symptoms like diarrhoea and abdominal pain, are caused by sensitive nerves and result in inflammation in the intestinal walls. For example, we usually all pass the same amount of gas a day (about 14 times, or 1 litre total), but some of us sense discomfort from that gas more than others do.

■ **Psychological responses:** Food aversions can develop if, say, a person had a bad vomit-inducing shellfish dinner one night. The response would be to associate the shellfish with the painful aftereffects and avoid it.

Of course, there are a number of extreme-end gastrointestinal problems like infections, parasites (worms are the world's most successful weight-loss technique – but we don't recommend the *Fear Factor* diet), and violent and even lethal allergic reactions to food. The point is that we all may have degrees of intolerance in ways we may not even recognize. And we need to start listening to what our small intestine is trying to tell us about what we eat. Once you recognize that the general sense of 'feeling off' can be caused by the foods you eat, you can identify – and work to eliminate, reduce or substitute – the substance that makes your gut twist like an animal balloon.

Here, we'll look at how inflammation happens at the gut level, and then, in the next chapter, how that can lead to inflammation at the total-body level.

FACTOID

For those of you who've stayed up wondering, here's the reason why your gas may smell and other people's gas may not: Think of your body as a refrigerator. If you let food sit in there, it's going to smell after a while. In your body, sulphur-rich foods like eggs, meat, beer, beans and cauliflower are decomposed by bacteria to release hydrogen sulphide – a smell strong enough to flatten a bear. Avoiding these foods is the ideal solution, but when stinky gas persists, the best solutions are leafy green vegetables and probiotics (specifically lactobacilli GG or Bifidus Regularis), which work like baking powder in your fridge to reduce odour.

Inflamed Gut: The Intestinal Firefights

At the intestinal level, foods can cause inflammation of your intestinal wall through such things as allergies, bacteria or other toxins. When food incites inflammatory responses in your gut, it's as if a grenade has been launched throughout your digestive system (see Figure 4.1 opposite). Then in response to this already damaging grenade, your body tosses more grenades to create an apocalyptic digestive War of the Worlds. The effect is that the more inflammation we have in our intestines, the more toxins can enter our bloodstream.

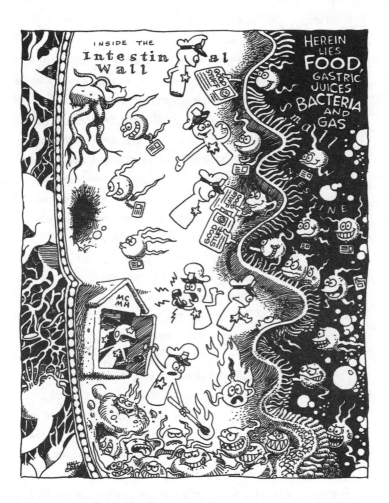

Figure 4.1 Internal Conflict

Food and toxins continually line the frontier of our intestines. Good foods slip through to provide us with nutrition, but combatants stimulate an aggressive response from local immune cells. The resulting inflammation causes swelling, gas and belly cramps.

During this firefight along the digestive border, your body perceives a foreign intruder and assigns its special forces – mast cells and macrophages – to eliminate the culprit. These are the cells that start an immune-response process throughout your body by ingesting foreign elements and alerting the rest of your body's protecting cells that intruders have entered the area. This causes your whole body to start firing away at these foods and at innocent bystanders – and thus causes inflammation in your bloodstream. In that way, eating unhealthy food is really like having a chronic infection that triggers an immune response, which then causes inflammation.

One of your body's goals is to get glucose into your brain cells – to feed those brain cells so that they can function. But inflammation in your body prevents sugar from getting to those cells, so you end up wanting more glucose and eating more sugary foods, which then increase inflammation and starts the whole cycle again.

While we should be concerned about decreasing our body fat, we should also concentrate on decreasing our body's inflammatory response so we become more efficient in managing potential complications of our waist size. There's some genetic component to inflammation (some us have more than others, and smokers tend to have higher levels of inflammation than non-smokers). Most important, the process of gaining weight is often a process of inflammation.

YOU-reka!
When you decrease your body's inflammatory response, you will decrease your weight and waist as well.

The more inflammation you have, the less efficiently you use your food calories, and the worse you feel. The worse you feel, the more bad foods you eat to try to make yourself feel better. The more bad food you eat, the less well you can respond to the normal stresses of life, and the more inflammation you experience. And the more inflammation you have, the higher your risk of developing:

- diabetes
- high blood pressure
- bad cholesterol numbers
- and all of the other conditions that contribute to your increase in size and your decrease in health.

FACTOID
Probiotics like lactobacillus GG or Bifidus Regularis repopulate your small intestine's bacteria with healthy bacteria, especially after a course of antibiotics. The good bacteria calm down the dangerous ones – meaning that they can help you have less gastrointestinal irritation, less gas and less risk of an inflammatory uncivil war breaking out.

Plain and simple: inflammation ages your body by making your arteries less elastic and by increasing atherosclerosis (the rusting of blood vessels). Inflammation also makes it more likely that your DNA will be damaged, and a cell will become cancerous. And it increases your risk of infections. If the inflammatory mediators are fighting in the arteries, they can't be defending elsewhere, and this situation increases the risk that your body will turn on itself, causing an autoimmune disease in which you attack your own tissues (for example, some forms of rheumatoid arthritis and thyroid disease).

Inflammation stresses your body.

Inflammation fattens your body.

Obesity isn't just a disease of doughnuts. Obesity is a disease of inflammation.

As we travel through the rest of our digestive journey, we'll be stopping at three digestive landmarks to see how foods influence inflammation and how inflammation influences fat:

Your Motorway of Food: Your Small Intestine

This approximately 20-foot-long organ (it's about three times your height) serves as your second brain, deciding which foods agree with your body and which foods cause your body to rebel like school children with a supply teacher.

FACTOID

We have two main sources that power nature's rear-propulsion system. Gas comes from the air we swallow (20 per cent) and the digestion of foods by bacteria in our intestines (80 per cent). These bacteria love digesting sugars, fibre or milk (if you're lactose-deficient). The result is lots of gas made up of carbon dioxide, nitrogen and methane (which – *duck!* – is flammable). You can reduce swallowing air by avoiding cigarettes, gum and carbonated beverages, or by eating and drinking more slowly.

Your Car Park of Fat: Your Omentum

The omentum, which is located next to your stomach, serves as your primary storage facility of fat, where you park some or (in really bad cases) all the excess foods you eat. Ideally, the car park is empty. But as we gain weight, some of our bellies are housing large amounts of fat. Most important, the omentum serves as our body's ultimate stress gauge:

YOU-reka!

As we'll explain in a moment, bigger bellies indicate higher levels of inadequately managed chronic stress – which causes chronic levels of inflammation.

Your Mail Sorting Office: Your Liver

Your liver is the second-heaviest organ in your body (the largest, your skin, is actually twice as heavy) and is your body's metabolic machine. Your liver works a lot like a sorting office, taking in all the incoming mail (in terms of nutrients and toxins), sorting it, detoxifying it and then shipping it off to different destinations for your body to use as energy.

While the three organs all play different roles, the upshot of their relationship is this: the small intestine initially processes your food, and your omentum helps store it. Inflammation occurs in your small intestine and omentum, but the big battle happens in your liver, where the mother of all inflammatory responses takes place. That's the one that makes you store fat – and experience the unhealthy effects of it.

Yes, we know that in-your-gut physiology isn't always pretty, but we want you to keep in mind our main gut goal: by understanding how food travels through this leg of your digestive system, you'll be able to identify the foods that will help you reduce harmful and weight-related inflammation. When you do that, you'll have signed a digestive peace treaty that can end the war on your waist.

Gathering Intelligence

They say that a woman thinks with her heart, and a man thinks with his personal periscope, but when it comes to sheer anatomy, the organ closest to your brain isn't the one that flutters over a midnight serenade or the one that tingles over a lingerie catalogue. It's the one that coils through your gut like a sleeping python.

From a purely physiological standpoint, your small intestine functions as your second brain. It contains more neurons than any organ but your brain (and as many as your spinal cord), and the physical structure of the small bowel most resembles that of the brain. In addition, after your brain, your small intestine experiences the greatest range of emotions – in this case, your feelings manifest themselves in the form of gastrointestinal distress. In your brain, you react to actions: you feel love when your spouse holds your hand; annoyed when he forgets an anniversary. Your small intestine does the same thing. It reacts to foods that enter its pathway, depending on their anti- or pro-inflammatory effect. Your foods dictate whether your small intestine feels mild annoyance (a little bloating), anger (gas), stubbornness (constipation) or all-out temper tantrums (a thar-she-blows case of diarrhoea).

Of course, you're the one who decides what foods you'll eat, but your small intestine works like an under-cover agent – gathering information about all the nutri-ents and toxins that enter your body.

Your small intestine feels. Your intestine thinks. And your intestine performs a critical job during digestion: It

Why Some People Stall

We'd like to think that our bodies work like cars – press the accelerator to go faster, tap the brakes to slow down. But our body's metabolic switches don't quite work that way: We may not gain or lose weight at the rate we expect to. When we have inflammation, our bodies are less efficient, meaning that we burn more calories – as a way to protect you, even as you gain weight. As we lose weight and decrease inflammation, our bodies go back to being efficient, and we may not burn calories at the proportional rate at which we gained them. So when we eat the right foods and more efficiently metabolize them, weight also may stall temporarily – meaning you still may be heavy, but might not have as many health risks associated with the weight.

helps guide you in all of the decisions *you* make about eating, because it tells you which foods agree with your body and which ones don't. How does it do that? Through the absorption of those foods. Your small intestine has an absorptive surface area that's 1,000 times larger than its start-to-end length because of all of the accordion-like nooks, crannies and folds within it. Those spaces are where your body actually absorbs nutrients. So your intestinal absorption area isn't just 20 feet long; it's the equivalent of 20,000 feet long. No wonder you absorb so much of what you eat. When you have inflammation in the wall of your small intestine (through a food allergy or intolerance), it dramatically cuts down on that absorptive surface area – from about 2 million square centimetres to 2,000 square centimetres – because of swelling and poisoning of the functional surface cells. And if the intestine can't absorb nutrients, you experience an upset stomach and diarrhoea.

While we're all familiar with those overt, emergency intestinal crises, our intestinal emotions also influence us in ways we don't normally associate with food. The reason we may feel groggy or lack energy could be because our intestines are trying to tell us we're choosing the wrong foods. If you pulled out the small intestines of your entire family and laid them out in the back garden to compare them (latex gloves, please), you'd see that they all look alike; they're the classic, wormy tubes that wind throughout your gut. In terms of basic physiology, we all have the same intestines, just as we all have the same basic brain structure. But just as all of our brains don't function the same way even though we have the same parts, our intestines don't function the same way either.

YOU-reka!

Our intestines are as different as our smiles, as our laughs, as our political views, as our fetishes. A particular food can make one person feel energized and make another person feel as lethargic as a rag doll.

Anatomically, your intestinal wall is Clint Eastwood tough. With more than a trillion bacteria living in your intestines at any given time (most of them helpful, but at least 500 species of which are potentially lethal), your body protects itself with a fortified infrastructure to keep the bacteria out of your bloodstream. But your body – though it relies on that Fort Knox–like wall – has to have a way to give clearance to authorized visitors. That is, it needs to allow nutrients to get through the wall to your bloodstream so you can use food as energy to keep your organs functioning, to go to work, to prise the kid's fingers from the panicked frog's leg. (One of the ways this penetration system works is through bile, which tricks the wall's security so fats can get through to the bloodstream.) This selection of what stays in your intestines and what can cross the line is one of the least understood anatomical processes, but it's part of the inflammatory battle that plays out daily in your body. When your intestinal wall is inflamed, some unauthorized visitors get in.

Essentially, alien bacteria are living in your intestines, trying to get into your bloodstream to multiply (which is their goal) and cause havoc, but they're being fought at the intestinal wall by those who guard it. (Your gastrointestinal tract, but especially your intestines, is one of three places where your body interacts with the external world; your skin and lungs being the other two.) In your small intestine, your mast cells and macrophages, which are part of your immune system, serve as the bowel brigade, fighting alien invaders.

When foods enter the small intestine and are transported across the intestinal wall, they're met by this bowel brigade border patrol, which screens the nutrients. The bowel brigade lets the food through because it has an

Milking It

If you suffer from a milk allergy, it can make your gut feel like a washing machine on the rinse cycle. Here are some ways you can help manage it:

- Milk's one of the easiest ingredients to substitute in baking and cooking by using an equal amount of either water, fruit juice or soya or rice milk.
- Watch out for hidden sources of dairy. For example, some brands of canned tuna fish and other non-dairy products contain casein, a milk protein.
- In restaurants, tell your waiter about your allergy. Many restaurants put butter (which comes from milk) on steaks and other food after they've been grilled or prepared to add extra flavour, but you can't see it after it melts.
- Some ingredients seem to contain milk products or derivatives but actually don't. These are safe to eat if you have a lactose allergy: cocoa butter, cream of tartar and calcium lactate.

By the way, there's a higher ethnic predominance of lactose intolerance in those of non-European origin. It's just another example of how genes – not willpower – help dictate what you can and cannot eat.

authorized ID card – it's food, and your body wants it. But if it's the wrong kind of food, or if it's got some toxins with it, your bowel brigade responds by calling in more mast cells and setting off time-released bombs throughout your intestines. This is where the inflammation firefight starts. The result? Pain, gas, nausea or general discomfort.

Why is this crucial? Not just because of the initial inflammatory reactions, but for the role it plays in your eating emotions (your small bowel is your second brain, and 95 per cent of your body's serotonin, which is a feel-

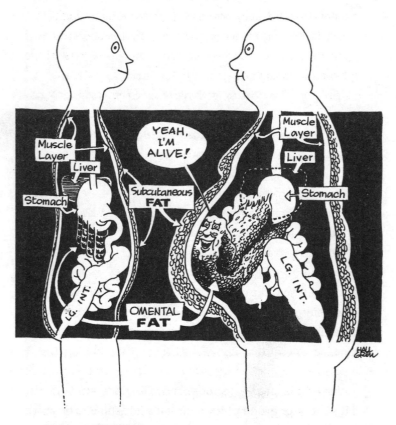

Figure 4.2 Belly Up

Not all fat is skin-deep. Deep down under your muscles, the omentum drapes off the stomach like stockings on a hanger. As we store fat, the omentum wraps around to give us the dreaded beer belly.

good hormone, is in your gut). How you feel influences how you eat, and how you eat influences how you feel. When you eat food that makes you feel bad, you self-medicate with food that may make you feel good in the short term but will actually contribute to both inflammation and weight gain. Ultimately, when you're caught in a cycle of feeling bad and eating worse, you'll create a chemical stress response in your body – one that's handled by your car park of fat.

The Storage of Stress in Your Belly

The best way to tell how stressed you are: take a look how much belly fat you have. The larger your waist, the higher your stress.

Along the intestinal motorway, the car park for fat that is your omentum looks like a stocking draped over a hanger (the stomach is the hanger), but changes depending on how many calories you're storing (see Figure 4.2). In a person with little omentum fat, the stomach looks as if it has nylons hanging off it – thin, permeable, with some webbing. But in a person with a lot of omentum fat, the fat globules are so fat that there's no netting or webbing whatsoever.

Genetics certainly helps dictate whether you're going to have a full car park (by having lots of belly fat) or an empty one. But your lifestyle – in terms of stress – often plays a bigger role in deciding whether you'll have large amounts of belly fat or not. Here's how it works:

Historically, mankind has had two types of stresses. The first kind is the immediate soil-your-loincloth stress (in other words, the dinner-seeking sabre-toothed tiger is closing in fast). In that fight-or-flight scenario, your body produces the neurotransmitter norepinephrine to speed your heart rate, breathing and 100-metre-dash time to the cave. When that happens, the last thing you're thinking about is grilling up some tubers on the campfire, so your hunger levels are squashed. That's because your body inhibits the peptide NPY during periods of acute stress (it's why exercise cuts appetite, because your body senses that you're in acute stress). So high levels of stress work in favour of your waist: They take away your appetite and speed up your metabolism.

The second kind of stress that early man faced was the chronic struggle brought on by drought and famine. In contrast to the 30 or 40 seconds they sweated over tiger fangs, our ancestors worried about survival all the time, and their bodies had to deal with chronic stress. When they faced famine, they sought out as many calories as they could, and their metabolism downshifted to help them conserve energy. While we don't deal with famine, we experience modern-day versions of chronic stress that make us seek out calories and then downshift our metabolism.

YOU-reka!

Our bodies respond by storing the excess energy to call upon during periods where there may not be enough food. Those extra calories are stored in the omentum – our abdominal fat depot – to have on hand in case we are denied food. The liver, which is the relay station for energy circulation in the body, has immediate access to this omental fat, unlike the cellulose cluttering up the back of our thighs.

When people are under stress, their bodies release high amounts of steroids into their bloodstream in the form of the hormone cortisol. In acute cases (the tiger or a car accident), steroids stick around briefly. But when you're under chronic stress (the drought or the nagging task), your body needs to find a way to deal with those high levels of cortisol. So your omentum clears the cortisol steroids; it has receptors that bind to them and can suck them out of the bloodstream. (Unfortunately, this doesn't necessarily reduce the stress level that you feel.) The steroids turbo-charge the ability of omentum to store fat, so your belly fat (and subsequent waist size) becomes the best surrogate indicator of how well you are really coping with stress – despite what your brain might be claiming. That uptake of steroids throws your body into metabolic disarray by making your omentum resistant to insulin so that sugar floats around without being absorbed and used appropriately by needy cells. This:

- chronically raises your blood sugar, which damages your tissues;
- supercharges your omentum with inflammatory chemicals that destabilize the delicate equilibrium of your hormones;
- forces your omentum to pump high-octane fat directly into your liver – causing your liver to make even more inflammatory chemicals.

The Fight against Inflammation

The liver – the organ that's responsible for your metabolism – receives its blood and nutrients from your gut. What it wants isn't the trans fat from the extra-large fries. It wants the other nutrients: the protein from the meat, the carbohydrates from the bun, the lycopene from the tomato, the calcium from the cheese. The liver is always on the job, processing munchies after midnight, as well as 5 a.m. coffee. Your liver takes every chemical in your body and processes it by binding it to a protein, transforming it into something the body can use.

So your poor overworked liver also gets the toxic trans fat directly from your intestines and from your omentum via that portal vein that feeds right into it. When your intestines send that convoy of fat pouring down into the vein, the liver sees it as a runaway train and tries to metabolize the foods. But in defending the body, additional inflammatory chemicals are released.

FACTOID

Preliminary studies in animals show that the scent of grapefruit oil – yes, just the scent – has an effect of reducing the appetite and body weight. Rats exposed to the scents for 15 minutes three times a week enjoyed the effect. The cause? It's unclear, but it may work through grapefruit oil's effects on liver enzymes. Grapefruit oil is widely available through aromatherapy shops and websites. As a bonus, try to eat a couple of grapefruit while you're searching.

In your liver, nutrients can be met by two substances: one bad, one good. Eating foods that stimulate your liver to release nuclear factor kappa B, or NF-kappa B, triggers a chain of events that causes the inflammation in your body and prevents the transport of glucose to your cells (and thus triggers hunger). Glucose (sugar) on the inside of cells stops hunger (in the specific satiety centre of the brain). But you can also eat foods that stop the inflammation riot or foods that stimulate the release of the do-good substances that have an anti-inflammatory effect. They're called PPARs (it stands for peroxisome proliferator-activated receptors, but we like to think of them as Perfectly Powerful Abdominal Regulators). The reason PPARs are so effective: once they're activated, they decrease glucose and insulin levels, as well as cholesterol and inflammation. Though we all have different genetic dispositions for levels of PPARs, PPARs aren't self-starters; they need to be activated by foods to work.

Now, if you look at PPAR and NF-kappa B at the cellular level, you can also see how they predispose us to obesity. Every human cell is run by DNA strands that carry blue-prints for future growth. When the DNA mutates, it makes our cells less able to reproduce themselves rapidly and accurately, so our bodies age. What makes that DNA break down? Yes, inflammatory responses in your body that cause oxidation (remember that this is your body's rusting process) – namely in the form of increasing NF-kappa B with inadequate PPAR levels to put out the inflammatory fires. How do we stop that mutation, that oxidation and that inflammation? By eating foods with antioxidant and anti-inflammatory properties – foods that we'll cover in the waist-management plan on page 242. These foods are particularly useful for those who are aging and unable either to exercise or to manage stress efficiently.

This is one of the primary battles you want to win – to calm your inflammation and decrease your fat storage through the regulation of these two chemicals and their allies. To quash those hooligans living in the NF-kappa B house, you need to increase the effects of the noble PPARs throughout your body.

The Stress Response: Putting it All Together

Today, we don't experience droughts or famine, but we do have high levels of chronic stress, whether it comes in the form of workload, relationship troubles or to-do lists that are longer than your arm. And our bodies respond the same way as our ancestors' bodies did. But the difference is that we have plenty of food at our disposal. Chronic stress triggers an ancient response of calorie accumulation and fat storage, so we end up continually upgrading the size of our omentum storage unit. Here's where the cycle of fat spins out of control:

- When you have chronic stress, your body increases its production of steroids and insulin, which …
- Increases your appetite, which …
- Increases the chance you'll engage in hedonistic eating in the form of high-calorie sweets and fats, which …
- Makes you store more fat, especially in the omentum, which …
- Pumps more fat and inflammatory chemicals into the liver, which …
- Creates a resistance to insulin, which …
- Makes your pancreas secrete more insulin to compensate, which …
- Makes you hungrier than a muzzled wolf, which …
- Continues the cycle of eating because you're stressed and being stressed because you're eating.

Interestingly, the more fat you store in your omentum, the more it reduces the effect of stress on your brain – it's your body's way of comforting you, assuring you that you'll be prepared during times of famine. It's why your omentum fat – the fat around your belly – isn't just an indicator of the size of your waist; it's also your own personal gauge of the size of your stress.

YOU Tips!

Let Food Fight the Fight

Your best weapon against fat isn't a do-it-yourself liposuction vacuum. It's food. Good food. Inflammation-reducing food. To reduce obesity-causing inflammation, you need to eat foods with nutrients that can do just that – either by having direct anti-inflammatory or antioxidant properties, or by stimulating the do-good PPARs or inhibiting the hooligan NF-kappa Bs. Antioxidants are often what gives a specific food its flavour, smell and colour. So eating more anti-inflammatory foods means eating more flavoursome and brightly coloured foods. (The foods you eat ought to be tasty; you can magnify a flavour by doubling up on it with two different food sources. For example, add sun-dried tomato bits to tomato sauce, or eat dried apples with apple sauce to bring out the flavour.)

Following is a list of nutrients that seem to have anti-oxidant and/or anti-inflammatory effects, and our

Is There Such a Thing as a Bad Food?

Fast-food franchise owners aren't the only ones who may say that there's no such thing as good or bad food – that it's just the volume of food that you eat. There are plenty of dietitians, nutritionists, doctors and food growers who believe the same thing. Our research leads us respectfully to disagree. Good, healthy foods satiate you, they decrease inflammation in your body, they decrease the tendency to yo-yo, they're nutrient-dense and they make you younger. Bad foods make you more hungry, increase inflammation in your body, make you feel sluggish, make it more likely you'll yo-yo, have few nutrients and make you older. After all, when you eat fries (no matter whether it's two fries or two bags), you're taking in calories that taste good, but have as much nutrient value as plywood. Good foods make waist management easier because they help keep you satisfied so that you never feel like gorging on nutrient-low and calorie-high foods. We call those good foods the YOU-th-FULL foods.

recommended doses. While they may not help you lose a ton of weight, they're known or thought to have anti-inflammatory effects, which will help you live healthier no matter what your weight.

Substances Known to Fight Inflammation

Omega-3 Fatty Acids: Omega-3 fatty acids – found in fish oils – seem to increase the number of PPARs, which will help reduce your inflammation. We recommend you get omega-3s in the form of three 4-ounce servings of fish per week or a 2-gram fish oil capsule a day or an ounce of walnuts a day. (Saturated fats, by the way, increase inflammatory properties, and trans fat undermines the effects of omega-3s.)

Green Tea: The thinking is that catechins in green tea inhibit the breakdown of fats and also inhibit production of NF-kappa B. Studies have found that drinking three glasses of green tea a day reduced body weight and waist circumference by 5 per cent in three months. It also increased metabolism (all non-herbal teas have substances that increase the metabolic rate).

Substances We Think May Fight Inflammation

Beer (in moderation, Tiger): The bitter compounds that come from hops derived from beer seem to activate PPARs in animal studies. But you have to get them in the form of only one drink a day. People who drink 21 8-ounce beers, or 21 glasses of wine, or 21 shots of whisky a week have a clear correlation predisposing them to belly fat, independent of all other risk factors.

Turmeric: A ginger-like plant that has curcumin as its active ingredient, turmeric seems to activate more PPARs to reduce inflammation. Just add the right dose – a pinch (1/8 of a teaspoon). Add any more and your food will taste like mustard.

Jojoba Beans (They are really seeds): They've been shown to tune up the system in the ways we want, like increasing good cholesterol levels and raising leptin levels to curb hunger. The supplement jojoba extract (the supplement simmondsin is also made from jojoba) seems to work by stimulating CCK. The dose is about 2.5 grams to 5 grams for most people (50 milligrams per kilogram of weight).

The Main Ingredients

Though the effect is not completely proven, there's some evidence that the following substances and ingredients have a meaningful anti-inflammatory effect:

Substance	Found In
Isoflavones	Soya beans, all soya products
Lignans	Flaxseed, flaxseed oil, wholegrains such as rye
Polyphenols	Tea, fruits, vegetables
Glucosinolates	Cruciferous vegetables such as broccoli and cauliflower, plus kale
Carnosol	Rosemary
Resveratrol	Red wine, grapes, red or purple grape juice
Cocoa	Dark chocolate
Quercetin	Cabbage, spinach, garlic

Drink Coffee

Coffee is a good source of polyphenols and is a great low-calorie fluid when you have cravings. You can drink de-caffeinated versions to avoid the side effects. The second-biggest source of antioxidants? Bananas, which have seven times less than coffee.

Go through the Process of Elimination

To change the way you feel, the way you process food and the way you store fat is to get at the root of the system: You need to work out what foods may be causing you gastrointestinal trouble, no matter how subtle your symptoms may be. The best way to do that is through the food-elimination test. What you'll do is completely eliminate certain groups of foods for at least three days in a row. (Sometimes, the elimination of a food takes two or more weeks to show its benefits in how you feel.) During that time, take notes about all the different ways you feel: your energy levels, fatigue and how often you go to the toilet. Take notes when you eliminate foods and when you reintroduce them – that way you'll really notice what changes make you feel worse or better.

Here's the order we suggest: wheat products (including rye, barley and oats), dairy products, refined carbohydrates (especially sugar), saturated and trans fats, and artificial colours (which are tough to get rid of because they're in everything). While the experiment will help you identify your personal digestive destructors, it has an added benefit: Eliminating a group of foods for several days at a time will help train your body to eat smaller portions all the time.

Get Moving after a Big Meal

If you've made a mistake and gorged on a tub's worth of food, make your body work in your favour. Stay awake for a few hours and take a 30-minute walk to help your body with the breakdown of nutrients and so that it uses the food for energy, rather than storing it as fat. Once the calories are in your stomach, don't try to vomit; vomiting can damage your stomach, burn your oesophagus, and even discolour your teeth if you do it enough. Also, don't eat sweets after gorging, because sweets will increase insulin and help deposit excess calories in your belly.

Pick Your Poison

High amounts of sucrose (sugar) cause inflammation; you can reduce the effect by using alternative sweeteners. Besides causing sudden spikes in blood sugar, foods with high sugar content have high calorie content, and if not burned off or used as fuel, those calories will be stored as fat. While some sweeteners are low- or no-calorie, there is a downside: sweeteners found in diet soft drinks, in diet foods and on restaurant tables next to the sugar packets go unrecognized by the brain. They're essentially invisible to your brain's satiety centres, so it doesn't count them as real food and still desires to be fulfilled by calories somewhere else. There's no clear-cut proof on the effects of these sweeteners – either on a health level or on a weight-loss level – but we do know one thing: prehistoric man wasn't putting Splenda in his water. Artificial sweeteners, while lacking calories, may have side effects like intestinal problems and headaches. If you're having a hard time losing weight or don't feel well, these are some of the first things to cut out, even though they can be an alternative to high-calorie sugars.

Chapter 5

TAKING A FAT CHANCE

How fat ruins your health

Diet Myths

- Thin people are automatically healthier than fat people.
- A fat is a fat is a fat. All fat is equally damaging.
- Your ideal blood pressure is anything less than 140/90.

It doesn't matter whether you're just trying to shave a few inches from your waist or trying to morph your slushy belly into an ice-hard one, the fact remains: it's hard to forget about body fat. You see it when you get dressed, get washed and get jiggy. You feel it when you sit down, when you walk upstairs, when you bend over to lick the last cake crumbs off the plate. And if you're a person who's struggled with weight for a lifetime, you likely stress about fat more than you stress about money, relationships or anaesthesia-free colonoscopies.

Fat is constantly right in our faces. And on our minds. And wrapped around our necks and arms. And hanging from our bellies. But you know what?

Often, we forget about fat. We eat a lot of food at one meal and go back to do it right again – because we don't see the health risks in the same way we see a slightly larger chin in the mirror. Now that our digestive journey is over, and you've learned how fat is stored, it's time to explore what that excess stored fat can do – to your heart, to your arteries, to your entire body.

Most of us assume that you have to be as skinny as a coaxial cable to be healthy, but the truth is that plenty of so-called thin people are less fit and less healthy than so-called heavy people.

YOU-reka!

That's right: it's actually better to be fat and have few risk factors for bad health than it is to be thin and have a high number of health-related risk factors. Now, that's not to say we're ordering a round of French fries for everyone. When all else is equal, carrying extra fat will more likely increase your risk of heart attacks, strokes and diabetes. But our point is that we want you to stop thinking about pounds and pounds only; we'd rather you start thinking about the numbers that really matter – especially to your husbands, wives, children, parents and friends. The real story of your body isn't measured by scales or wolf whistles. It's measured by your waist size – and what fat does inside your blood and arteries.

What Fat's Got to Do with It

Here's how many of us assess our health: if the pain's not severe enough to call the doctor, then we tough it out, go on our way and write off most of our general feel-bad symptoms to fatigue, stress, age or the tub of ice cream we downed during *CSI*. The problem with that approach? You're probably more in tune with the autumn television schedule than you are with your own body. Of course, if you're overweight, the extra fat is sure to manifest itself in some outward side effects like lack of energy or lack of self-esteem. But many of the risk factors associated with carrying too much fat don't have any outward symptoms at all – meaning that the only way to tell whether being overweight is threatening your life is by taking a microscope underneath the flub and chub and focusing on what's happening at your body's most core levels.

Of course, you know that fat lives on your hips, but it also lives in your blood. If you were to take a vial of blood and let it sit (we don't recommend doing this at home), you'd see a layer of clotted cream that would rise to the top of the vial, rather like tiramisu. That's fat. How did it get there? (Half credit if your answer was tiramisu.) It's absorbed via your intestines. But the key player is the omentum. And why should we care about that organ that sounds like it's missing the letter *m*? Because the omentum can store fat that is quickly accessible to the liver (meaning it can cause lousy cholesterol and triglyceride levels to rise) and also sucks insulin out of circulation (making your blood sugar rise) – meaning that this cream-converted fat sets up shop in the omentum and puts your organs within very close striking distance of a hammer.

See, fat is like property: it's all about location, location, location. We all have three kinds of fat: fat in our bloodstream (called triglycerides), subcutaneous fat (which lies just underneath the skin's surface) and that omentum fat. (The fourth fat, of course, is the fat in food.) As you remember from the last chapter, the omentum is a fatty layer of tissue located inside the belly that hangs *underneath* the muscles in your stomach (it's why some men with beer guts have hard-as-keg bellies – their fat is underneath the muscle).

Because this omentum fat is so close to your solid organs, it's their best energy source. (Why go to the petrol station on the other side of town when there's a station at the next corner?) Think of the omentum fat as the obnoxious lorry on a crowded motorway – elbowing out the stomach, pushing away other organs and claiming all the space for itself (see Figure 5.1).

What's most interesting – and encouraging – is that as soon as you make physiological changes to your omentum, your body starts seeing effects. That is, once your body senses it's losing that fat, then your body's blood-related numbers (cholesterol, blood pressure, blood sugar) start travelling in the healthy direction – within days, before you even notice any kind of physical sign of weight loss (especially when you consider that the size of your omentum is impossible to measure without a CT scan).

In addition, the fat released from the omentum travels to your liver rapidly and constantly as opposed to the

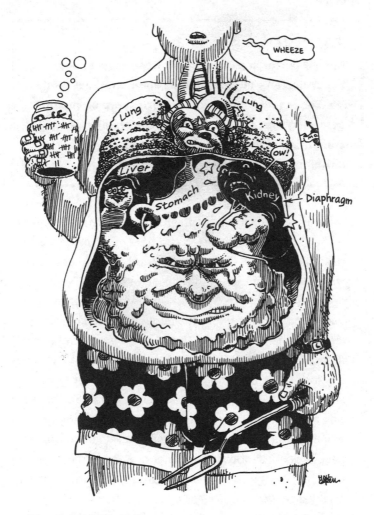

Figure 5.1 Belly Bully

The omentum greedily bullies surrounding structures out of the way. The squished diaphragm and lungs make breathing difficult, and the squashed kidney and its blood supply secrete hormones to raise the blood pressure in an effort to fight back.

FACTOID

Recent research shows that coffee doesn't cause hypertension – but caffeinated sugar and diet drinks do. The reason? It may be the corn syrup or caramel colouring that's responsible for the change. It's something to keep in mind when considering caffeine as a potential waist-control drug.

more patient fat on your thighs. The processed material is then shipped to the arteries, where it is linked to health risks like high LDL (lousy) cholesterol. The other problem with omentum fat is that it secretes very little adiponectin, which is a stress- and inflammation-reducing chemical that's related to the hunger-controlling hormone leptin. When you have less fat, you secrete more adiponectin, which produces a product that reduces inflammation. But more importantly, higher levels of adiponectin are related to lower levels of fat. So the more omentum fat you have, the less fat-regulating adiponectin you'll produce. Those who have low levels of adiponectin have abdominal obesity, high blood pressure, high cholesterol and other risk factors associated with coronary artery disease.

Those are the reasons why the fat in your thighs doesn't matter as much to your health as does omentum fat (even if it matters for your bikini pride), and they help explain why omentum fat (or an 'apple' body shape) is more harmful than subcutaneous fat (like thigh fat, which gives you a 'pear' shape). Subcutaneous fat isn't supplying a feeding tube to the rest of your vital internal organs, and it's not messing up the levels of substances in your blood that are being supplied to your vital organs.

The closer your waist is to ideal, the healthier your arteries and your immune system will be. The healthier your arterial and immune systems, the longer – and better – you'll live. And the more energy you'll have every day.

Highways to Health

Before you know what's inside your arteries, you need to know how they're structured – so you can see what kind of damage they can sustain and what kind they can't. Made up of three layers, your arteries are the monorails of your body – they transport blood throughout your body and deliver nutrients to all of your organs.

Inner layer: The innermost layer of your arteries (the intima) comes in contact with blood; it's slippery like Teflon so blood can easily flow through. This normally smooth layer helps protect the muscular middle layer (the media) and is the layer most susceptible to attacks from outside sources.

Middle layer: The middle layer of your arteries supports the entire arterial structure by working a little like a hand squeezing a hose or a boa constrictor squeezing a neck.

When you're depressed or anxious, the layer can constrict, narrowing the amount of space where blood can flow through (the lumen). But it also has an advantage; it can release tension by dilating (the hand releasing the hose) to pull the Teflon layer outwards and open up *more* space in the part of the artery where blood flows – say, when you exercise. When that happens, it allows more red cells, oxygen and other nutrients through. You feel more energetic when that layer functions like it did when you were nine years old.

Outer layer: The outer layer (the adventitia) shields the artery from the rest of your body like sausage casing; it holds the artery together from the outside.

Under normal circumstances, the inner layer is lined with delicate cells, and blood runs freely. Think of the structure as a tile wall – it's a smooth wall made up of individual tiles connected together with little gaps throughout. In the tile wall, you have white gooey grout; in the artery, you have tight junctions holding the cells together.

Now, in your arteries, that wall will stay tight unless something comes along and starts chipping away at the junctions between those smooth cells. The most damaging tile buster – high blood pressure – is the arterial sledgehammer. But plenty of other pickaxes can chip away at the arterial lining: cholesterol, nicotine, high levels of blood sugar, stress, anger and about 40 other smaller risk factors, primarily stemming from lifestyle choices you make. The effect? They chip away and cause little nicks in the intima of your arteries, and those injuries trigger the anatomical starter's pistol. The race to destroy – and repair – your arteries is on.

The Effects of Fat

For years, you've been used to looking down at a scale's needle to determine your health. Wrong needle. What you need: a needle in the hands of someone who can draw your blood. With results from a simple blood test, you'll find out what your current settings are and then be equipped with the data you need to take steps that will reset the settings to the factory originals.

Blood Pressure

High blood pressure still reigns as the leading cause of heart attack, stroke, heart failure, kidney failure and impotence. While most of your other blood numbers reveal levels of substances inside your blood, your BP gauges how your blood travels through your body. Simply, blood pressure refers to the amount of force exerted by your blood on your arterial walls as it passes through. It's measured through the systolic pressure (the pressure being exerted when the heart contracts; the top number) and the diastolic pressure (the pressure on your arteries when your heart is at rest).

Now, if the force of that pumping is too high, it'll gouge holes in that smooth inner lining of your arteries (see Figure 5.2), causing those nicks in the tile wall that trigger a chain reaction of grouting, then destructive inflammation and clotting (which we'll discuss in detail below). Think of it as the beating of a bongo: treat your arterial walls with a nice steady rhythm – let your blood *tap tap tap* them; not *pound pound pound* them. (Blood pressure fluctuates throughout the day; the goal is to have your total BP picture under control.)

Certainly, many factors can make your blood pressure soar (stress, high levels of the mineral sodium, lack of the mineral calcium or potassium from not enough fruits and vegetables, lack of physical activity). But it's also clear that being overweight leads directly to high blood pressure. This happens in part when the kidneys, squashed by fat, feign death unless they are fed with a higher blood pressure. (Your kidneys are the organ primarily responsible for regulating blood pressure.)

Luckily, you can reduce your blood pressure quickly and dramatically by addressing your waist issues. Losing 10 per cent of the weight you've gained since you were 18 (that's only four pounds if you've gained 40) can result in a decrease of 7 mmHg (stands for millimetres of mercury to measure the partial pressure of a gas) from your systolic number and 4 mmHG from your diastolic one. The message is clear: drop your waist and you'll drop your BP.

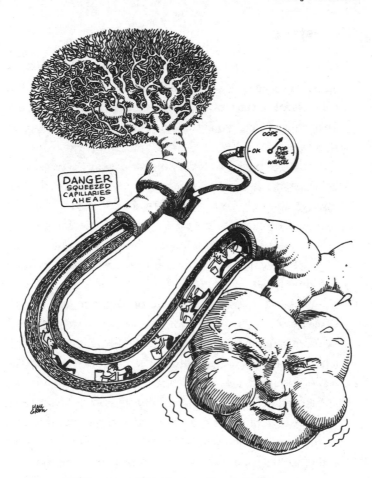

Figure 5.2 Pressure Situation

With hypertension, the arteries squeeze down so tightly that the heart struggles to keep the blood moving forward. To compensate, the heart gets too thick, like a muscle-bound weight lifter. It becomes so stiff that it loses flexibility and can't relax. If it can't relax, blood has trouble travelling through the arteries, and the resulting high blood pressure damages the arteries.

Cholesterol

Hear the word cholesterol and you're likely to think of eggs, heart attacks and a mandate from your doctor. But cholesterol is part of your body's arterial repair kit; it's designed to help you, though it doesn't always happen that way.

Let's go back to those nicks in your arterial wall. Whether it's BP, nicotine or too many cheese curls that damage the wall, your body gets angrier than a chained-up bull – because it doesn't want the middle lining of the artery exposed to blood. So your body hires a handyman to patch up your nicks with grout, to cover the wounds in the inner lining.

What's that grout? Cholesterol, but not just any ol' cholesterol.

Your handyman – let's call him Les – carries two things: a bucket of grout and a spatula. The grout can come in the form of lousy cholesterol, which is carried by low-density lipoprotein (LDL). It's big and puffy, and prone to breaking up and scattering bits of cholesterol when it hits the walls of the artery. When your LDL levels are too high to begin with (maybe from your diet or from your heredity), and then you nick the inner lining of one of your arteries, Les goes crazy and slaps on more and more and more grout. He starts covering up the damage with the bad cholesterol – loads and loads of bad cholesterol.

But look inside Les's tool belt. He's got a spatula that takes premium-grade grout in the form of cholesterol carried on high-density lipoprotein (it's the healthy HDL cholesterol). Compact and powerful, the spatula works with this slick stuff to take the extra gunk away.

Now, if you have too much of that LDL grout and not enough premium-version HDL grout (from not eating enough of the right kinds of foods and fats, not getting enough physical activity, or not having enough female hormones – yes, even men have them), it can lead to a chain of events that has potentially heart-stopping outcomes. We'll call it fat's domino effect.

Domino 1: Having too much bad cholesterol not only means you'll have too much junk (plaque) in your arteries. It also means that LDL cholesterol will get into the middle layer of your artery. That cholesterol in the middle layer acts like a drunk fan with courtside seats, making the environment much more hostile than it's used to being. The presence of LDL cholesterol in that middle layer stimulates the immune system to attract white-cell protectors to try to smooth out and calm down the rotten cholesterol.

Domino 2: Those white blood cells, in turn, spill some of their toxic contents that normally attack infections – and that causes generalized inflammation.

Domino 3: The toxic contents and cholesterol are soaked up by scavenger cells, building up blister-sized spaces in the walls of your arteries. They're called foam cells – and they increase the size of the plaque, or grout, even more to make the artery surface rougher.

Domino 4: Sensing something's wrong, your body responds with more inflammation, creating bulges and potholes in the wall, often in the area of weakness, where the initial nick was and a scar was trying to form over the dangerous plaque. If that plaque ruptures into the middle of your blood vessel, the next domino falls.

Domino 5: These rough patches in the wall then attract sticky blood platelets to form clots in your arteries. Normally, platelets are good (they help form scabs to heal wounds). But when they hit that rough patch in your arterial wall, they grab the lining and form a big clot on top of irritated, inflamed plaque. And this brings in more clotting proteins to the area that act to cement the platelets in place.

Domino 6: All of this gunk piles up faster and faster, and the inside of the arteries becomes so inflamed that the platelets and clots fill the entire artery.

YOU-reka!

This ruptured plaque process take minutes rather than decades, so you can influence its likelihood today by making the right choices about food.

Domino 7: The blood can't get through the artery, and nourishment to the heart is shut off.

Game Over: The chain reaction triggers a heart attack (or, depending where the process happens, causes a stroke, memory loss, impotence, wrinkled skin or any number of health problems that happen when blood flow malfunctions).

As you can see, it's not the cholesterol by itself that's so bad; it's not having high enough levels of healthy and/or low enough lousy cholesterol to thwart the process before it even begins. And it's not doing things like normalizing your blood pressure and blood sugar to help decrease the chance of developing nicks in the first place.

While genetics dictates some of your cholesterol level, your physical activity levels and poor foods choices – trans and saturated fats, simple sugar and too many calories – really dictate whether Les carries the right amount and kind of grout or moves the spatula fast enough to make for a nice, clean wall.

Blood Sugar

Blood sugar is another substance that can nick your arteries if levels are too high. You may think your level is normal, but most blood sugar levels are recorded when you've fasted. Having 'normal' levels for fasting (under 100 milligrams per decilitre, abbreviated 100 mg/dl) and for after meals (under 140 mg/dl) is important. Why? Because there's a good chance that even with normal blood sugar levels, your blood sugar may rise significantly throughout the day as you eat. Studies show that men with a waist of 40 inches or more have 12 times the risk of getting diabetes compared with men with a waist smaller than 35 inches. For women, having a 37-inch waist is that much riskier than having a 32½-incher. (The most sensitive way to diagnose diabetes is to measure the blood sugar fasting, and again two hours after taking 75 grams of sugar – to see how your body can deal with the sugar.)

Many people think that diabetes is a purely genetic disease, and of course, it would be nice to blame Aunt Mabel for the medical condition, but it doesn't quite work that way. For type 2 diabetes (type 1 is the juvenile form), your environment (that is, your lifestyle, your behaviours, your macaroons) is a much more dominant trait than genetics.

Yes, type 2 diabetes is a genetic disease. That is, if you are a twin and have an identical twin who gets type 2 diabetes, you have the genetics for it. And it's a tough disease, too: diabetes ages you one and a half years for every year you live. For example, if you get it at age 30 and live to 60, you're not really 60. You have the energy and disability risks of a 75-year-old.

Here's how it works: insulin in your blood normally takes sugar and puts it into the cells, but in people with type 2 diabetes, the transfer of sugar into your muscle and fat cells is inhibited. While nice in coffee, that sugar in your blood chips away at your arterial wall by weakening the junctions between cells that form the surface lining of your arteries. Ultimately it allows holes to form in these junctions. By causing your insulin levels to go haywire and making proteins in your body less effective, sugar really behaves like nutritional cocaine.

Omentum fat (belly fat) contributes to type 2 diabetes by making it difficult to get glucose inside the cell and let insulin do what it does best: deliver glucose. Simply being overweight, especially having a waist greater than 37 inches (85 centimetres) for women and 40 inches (100 centimetres) for men, makes your body less sensitive to insulin; the insulin receptors on the cells don't allow insulin to transmit the message enabling glucose transport into the cells, leaving the glucose to float around in your blood. That omentum fat is also selfish; it uses up the insulin so it can't do its job (one study shows omentum fat sucks up a quarter of the insulin that passes through the blood supply).

So your blood sugar level remains high because the sugar isn't being admitted to your cells readily and thus isn't broken down properly, meaning that sugar will hang out in your blood like a truant skipping school and causing mischief.

So what? Well, having too much sugar in your blood is like having too much rain in a small pond – the flooding can cause damage for everything around it. Too much blood sugar can:

- Weaken the junctions between those smooth endothelial cells lining your arteries, making the Teflon-like lining more vulnerable to nicks.
- Increase the power of the hammer, to cause high blood pressure. (Sugar turns the hammer into a sledgehammer.)
- Cause your white blood cells to stop fighting infections, thus weakening your immune system.
- Trigger a chemical process in your red blood cells, which transport oxygen in your bloodstream, that causes the cells to want to hold onto oxygen more tightly. That keeps oxygen from getting to your tissues. When that happens, the glucose, like a lost puppy, attaches to whatever it can find – most likely, proteins

in your blood and tissues. These proteins deposit in tissues, leading to the development of cataracts, joint abnormalities and lung problems.

- Get into your nerves and cause a reaction that makes your nerves swell, become compressed and lose their ability to function – usually in the parts of your body furthest from your brain: your hands and feet.
- Flip off a switch in your small blood vessels. Normally your body automatically regulates the flow of nutrients into your small blood vessels. They sort of work on backup (like a generator for when the power goes out), so they can function even when your big vessels might be experiencing problems. But high levels of glucose turn off that automatic regulation – and let a little high blood pressure make more of those nicks and tears in the junctions between cells in your smaller blood vessels. This is like asking someone to use a sledgehammer to do the job of a jeweller's tool; it magnifies that effect and magnifies the size of the nick.

But here's the thing. You can control your genes if you want to. To keep blood sugar levels down, you should avoid foods with simple sugar and lousy aging fats (trans and saturated fats). And about 1,000 calories' worth of activity a week – about 30 minutes of walking a day and 20 minutes of the YOU Workout three days a week – causes your muscles to be so much more sensitive to insulin, which allows sugar to do its duty inside your cells, rather than cause havoc in your bloodstream. A little physical activity goes a long way.

Arterial Inflammation

When we think of our arteries and what can damage them, we tend to think of that clog: the hunk of junk that stops the flow of blood like a lemon seed in a straw. If there's a roadblock in the way, then there's no way for traffic to move through. But that's only one mechanism for closing off blood flow. The other occurs through the process of inflammation. Typically, inflammation in our bodies makes us think of things that swell *out* – like a sprained ankle, swollen gums or the shiner from the 2 a.m. bar brawl. But when it comes to arterial inflammation, you have to think about swelling *in*. In response to all that clotting action we talked about with LDL cholesterol, inflammation occurs in the middle layer of your arteries. As the middle layer swells, it pushes into the inner layer because the outer sausage layer doesn't give. That pushing into the inner layer reduces the size of the hole that blood can travel through (like drinking with a thinner straw).

One of the ways we determine potential cardiovascular risks is by measuring chemicals in the blood that signal inflammation. C-reactive protein (CRP) is one such chemical; elevated CRP indicates an inflammatory reaction somewhere in your body, from a sinus infection to gum inflammation. If it's high, your risk of heart disease is greater, because any significant inflammation in your body increases inflammation in your blood vessels.

Fat Chance: The Other Major Risks

We're not here to lecture you and pummel you with statistics about health risks. But to put fat in perspective, remember that it's an all-body risk factor – with implications everywhere. Even if your numbers in some health categories are perfect, you're not risk-free. Being overweight or obese leads to the following:

Higher Risk of Cancer

The inflammation resulting from omentum fat also causes dysfunction in the system that protects you from cancer. In fact, there's a direct correlation between waist size and an increased risk of hormonally sensitive tumours, such as breast cancer in women and prostate cancer in men. Fat contains an enzyme, aromatase, which converts adrenal hormones into a long-acting kind of oestrogen, which can cause increased breast cancer risk.

Higher Risk of Sleep Apnoea

Fat around your waist correlates with a thick neck, and that can obstruct your breathing (you're at higher risk if your neck size is more than 17 inches). In its benign form – snoring – you can still move air through your throat, but generate a kazoo sound that can cause permanent hearing loss and marital strife. In some cases, that obstruction worsens, until eventually no air can pass into the lungs for up to 10 seconds at a time. Fortunately, the body instinctively awakens prior to suffocation. As you get older, the tissue in your throat softens, and the area around your tonsils attracts fat. When you're asleep, and your muscles fully relax, the tissue collapses, so there's even less room in the back of your throat.

Sleep apnoea makes you miss out on deep, restorative REM sleep. This leads to frequent awakenings at night (though your spouse may know it, you'll probably never feel yourself waking), lack of sleep and daytime drowsiness. You're more likely to develop nick-causing high blood pressure (caused when your lungs hang on to carbon dioxide when you stop breathing) and, the bitter irony, you're more likely to get fatter because of it. That's because sleep apnoea is like a series of rear-end collisions – one accident after another. The lack of sleep makes you tired. You feel like you need more energy. You eat foods that give you quick energy but also have high sugar and fat. You get fatter. You continue to have sleep apnoea. And the cycle continues. (As an incentive to embrace a good eating plan, most people will lose fat first in their faces and throats; so with a waist reduction of a few inches you'll probably be able to prevent or reduce these sleep problems by 30 per cent early in your programme.)

Higher Risk of Joint Problems

While strong, your joints are like parents trying to squash constant whining; they can take only so much before they break down. Your knees are some of the most powerful joints in your body because you use them to both push off and absorb force. But they're also prone to wear and tear if they have to carry a heavier load (that is, more fat in your body) than they're designed to. When you gain 10 pounds of body weight, it feels more like a 30-pound weight to your knees while you're walking. When you walk upstairs, the 10 pounds of fat feel like 70 pounds to your knee joint. That extra weight makes you more vulnerable to developing joint-deteriorating conditions like osteoarthritis, which occurs when your joints get nicks in their smooth cartilage from bearing a load they're not designed to carry.

When you reduce your omentum fat and your waist size, you'll automatically reduce your risk in so many areas of your health. Even better, you'll have the potential to see dramatic reductions in risk factors.

YOU-reka!

When overweight people (with an average weight of 225 pounds) lose about 7.5 per cent of their body weight (about 17 pounds or four inches of waist size), they improve their HDL and LDL cholesterol levels, BP and blood sugar numbers by – get this – 20 per cent. That's nearly three times the benefit compared with percentage weight loss. Take the following steps to help you get there in terms of both inches and risk factors.

YOU Tips!

Know Your Fats

Fat in foods, like bosses, comes in two broad categories: those that are good for your well-being and those that want you to suffer. The strongest influence you can have on your levels of cholesterol (not to mention your waist size) is by watching what fats you're eating and what fats you're banishing from your life and your gut.

Above all, you want to avoid saturated and trans fats; a serving size should have no more than 4 grams of those two villains combined. They're the foods most associated with long-term weight gain and clogging your arteries. Essentially, bad fats are ones that are solid at room temperature: animal fat, butter, stick margarine, lard. Trans fat contains cross-linked hydrogen bonds, which make it stable for long periods of time at room temperature. Eating trans fat leads to abnormalities in cholesterol (decreasing your good and increasing your bad), as well as increasing inflammation and damaging your arterial cells, which makes you more prone to clotting. (By the way, trans fat was originally designed for candle wax, but the market died with the advent of electricity.) The value of trans fats is that they have a long shelf life; the average food manufacturer would love to make foods with healthy fats if they could have the one-year shelf life that they can get from the unhealthy fats.

The good fats, by contrast, are the ones that are liquid at room temperature but get thick when they get cold, like olive oil. They help raise your HDL levels to clear away the gunk. Far more important than the calories of fat is what fatty acids can do to your cell functions, and how they influence arterial function and inflammation.

Super (Youthful) Fats: Facilitate Spatula Action	Stupid (Aging) Fats: Cause the Clogs, Clump up the Spatula
Monounsaturated Fats. They come in two forms: omega-3 fatty acids and omega-6 fatty acids, in the form of fish (3s) and nut oils (3s and 6s). The omega-3s have been shown to improve arterial and brain function. They're found in olive oil, canola oil, fish oils, flaxseeds, avocados and nuts (especially walnuts). They've also been shown to reduce blood pressure and lipid levels when used in place of carbohydrates.

Bottom line: Make about 30 per cent to 40 per cent of your fats the monounsaturated variety. | **Trans Fat.** This is the fat that contains hydrogenated vegetable oil. It's the worst kind of fat and will stunt weight-loss efforts. Trans-fatty acids are in all kinds of food – especially when long shelf life is important – from buttered popcorn and biscuits to crisps and margarine.

Bottom line: Say no. Stay away from them the way you'd avoid motorways on Christmas Eve. Clog city. |

Super (Youthful) Fats: Facilitate Spatula Action	Stupid (Aging) Fats: Cause the Clogs, Clump up the Spatula
Polyunsaturated Fats. These are like monounsaturated except that they contain more than one unsaturated bond. They are usually present in vegetable oils and sesame oils. They may improve arterial and brain function, and will help keep up your satiety levels. **Bottom line:** Make 20 per cent to 40 per cent of your fats polyunsaturated.	**Saturated Fats.** Found in meats and dairy products, these fats will make you gain weight and clog your arteries. **Bottom line:** Limit saturated fat to lean sources like lean cuts of beef and low-fat dairy products. Aim for less than 4 grams of saturated fat per serving. Less than 20 grams, or less than 30 per cent of your daily allotment, should be from saturated and/or trans fats combined.

Note: The best oil to have in your home is extra-virgin olive oil or organic (or cold-press) canola oil. For cooking, you can also use sesame or groundnut oil. That's because their smoking point – that is, the temperature at which the fat burns – is very high. Cook beyond it, and you'll end up with a burned, charcoal flavour. Once heated, oils can become rancid and also can generate toxic chemicals, so you lose the major benefit of eating these usually healthy foods. Also, it's best to cook the food, rather than the oil. So don't heat the oil directly in the pan; instead, roll your food in the oil first and then heat the food so the oil does-n't become overheated.

Smoke points (in Fahrenheit) for Some Commonly Used Healthy Oils

Unrefined canola oil	225°
Unrefined sunflower oil	225°
Extra-virgin olive oil	320°
Virgin olive oil	420°
Sesame oil	410°
Grape-seed oil	420°
Refined groundnut oil	450°
Semi-refined sesame oil	450°

Clear It All Up

More and more evidence is showing that clog-free living is correlated with raising your amount of HDL to thwart the clot-triggering process. By raising your HDL, you increase the amount of healthy cholesterol that's available to clear away the lousy cholesterol. Things that have been shown to effectively raise HDL include:

- Consuming healthy fats found in olive oil, fish, avocados and walnuts.
- Walking or doing any physical activity for at least 30 minutes a day – no excuses.

- Taking niacin. Take 100 milligrams four times a day. Regular (and OTC) niacin is much cheaper than prescription niacin, and there seems to be a beneficial effect of extended-release doses. Sometimes higher doses are needed, in which case your doctor needs to peek at your liver function to ensure that you avoid the uncommon toxicity. To reduce flushing (feeling hot and light-headed), take an aspirin half an hour beforehand and take the niacin as you go to bed. Do not increase the dose above this level without talking to your doctor, and check with your doctor before using niacin at any dose if you have a history of liver problems.

- Taking vitamin B5 (pantothenic acid). We recommend a dose of 300 milligrams a day to decrease LDL and raise HDL with no side effects yet known.

- Having one drink of alcohol every night. You should not be drinking just to get your HDL up, but if you do drink alcohol, stick to one drink, and you may see some small beneficial effects.

- Substituting protein or monounsaturated fat in place of carbs. Recent research suggests that this can help reduce BP and modify lipid levels.

Just Say Yes to This Drug

If there were one magic pill for fighting fat and saving lives, the pharmaceutical industry would send everyone from scale makers to diet-book authors into bankruptcy. There's no pill that will do it all. (At least not yet.) But that doesn't mean you can't use drugs to improve your health and reduce your cardiovascular risk factors. Our recommendation – and the closest thing to a pill with mystical powers – comes in the form of two baby aspirin (162 milligrams total) a day. You need two rather than one, since many people are resistant to the lower dose. (There is no measurable increased risk of stomach problems in studies with this small increase in doses from 81 milligrams to 162 milligrams, and the reduction in heart attacks or ischaemic strokes goes from around 13 per cent to around 36 per cent.) Aspirin makes platelets less sticky and decreases inflammation that occurs to narrow the space where blood flows through your arteries. And it's been shown to reduce arterial aging and immune system aging, and that means decreasing your risk of everything from heart attack, strokes and impotence to colon, rectal and oesophageal cancers, and maybe even breast and prostate cancers. To reduce the gastric side effects, drink half a glass of warm water before and after taking the pill. (See your doctor if you have any history of serious bleeding, are taking blood thinners or do extreme sports.)

Have Regular Readings

Not just with your book club or by an astrologer. These regular readings are about tracking your health numbers. Instead of measuring your success through the scale, the real measurement – and test – of your success is seeing whether you've reduced your cardiovascular risk, as evidenced in the following test readings:

Blood Pressure: Optimum level is 115/76. Blood pressure readings can be variable, so have your BP taken in the morning, during the day and at night, as part of your normal activities (except for 30 minutes after exercise, when it will naturally be higher). Take the average of three readings to come up with your base number. After that, take readings every month to help you monitor your progress. (If BP is high, then you can track it daily.)

Lipid Profile Blood Test: Have one now to establish your baseline measurement, then have your blood analysed every other year so that you and your doctor can watch changes and make appropriate adjustments to your eating and/or drug plan.

HDL (healthy) cholesterol: You're at a low risk if your HDL is greater than 40 mg/dl. But like basketball players, the higher the better. In fact, if your HDL is over 100 mg/dl, the chances of having a heart attack or stroke related to lack of blood flow are smaller than the chance that a Hollywood celeb could walk through Marks and Spencer unnoticed. (Except in some extremely rare cases where HDL malfunctions inside the body, there has never been a heart attack or stroke due to lack of blood flow reported in the entire medical literature in a person with a functional HDL over 100.)

LDL (lousy) cholesterol: You're at a low risk if your LDL is less than 100 mg/dl. By the way, research shows that for all women, and for men over 65 years old, the LDL number isn't nearly as important as the HDL. So women and men over 65 don't need to obsess too much over LDL levels unless their HDL levels are too low.

Fasting blood sugar: Below 100 mg/dl.

C-reactive protein: Below 1 mg/dl.

Get a Lift

Muscle isn't just for rugby players and bouncers. Everyone benefits from adding some muscle to his or her body; in fact, adding some muscle will help lower your levels of blood sugar. The more muscle you have, the more you increase insulin receptivity – that is, the process by which insulin transports glucose into your cells. If you gain muscle and lose weight, you change the chemistry of your cell membranes so that you absorb more glucose throughout your body rather than having it stay in your blood. You add muscle by doing strength exercises (more coming up in the YOU Workout).

Stop Freebasing Sugar

One thing that causes blood sugar to spike is, uh, sugar. That is, straight, pure sugar – not eaten with any other substances like fat or protein around it. Though we recommend eating as few simple sugars as possible, if you do eat them, you should always be sure not to eat that chocolate bar by itself. Have a handful of nuts or some olive oil with bread first; that slows your stomach from emptying and will keep sugar levels from creating a pyrotechnical effect in your blood.

Go Chrome

Chromium, a mineral found in a variety of foods (especially mushrooms), seems to help control blood sugar. Taking 200 micrograms a day of the supplement chromium picolinate can help aid the uptake of insulin, to help your cells use blood sugar for fuel. Though the studies aren't definitive at this point, we recommend the supplement for waist – and blood sugar – control. Chromium increases your cells' sensitivity to insulin and is depleted by refined sugars, white flour and lack of exercise. One study showed users lost four pounds over 10 weeks compared with no pounds in a control group. You should take it with magnesium, which reduces low-grade inflammation that can be associated with insulin resistance. A dose of 600 micrograms of chromium has been shown to be effective for those with type 2 diabetes, but for others, stick to the recommended dose of 200 micrograms. Just because a little is good doesn't mean that taking a lot more is better. Taking too much chromium can hurt your kidneys.

Become Sensitive

Here's a tantalizing observation: cinnamon seems to have an insulin-like effect, enhancing the satiety centre in your brain while also reducing blood sugar and cholesterol levels. Just half a teaspoon a day can have some effect. Sprinkle it in cereal or on toast, or add it to a smoothie.

Get in the Zone

Studies show that meditation has a statistically significant reduction of risk factors for coronary heart disease, such as blood pressure and insulin resistance. Find a quiet room, take a few minutes, close your eyes and focus on one healthy word or phrase, like 'om' (or 'omega-3 fatty acids').

Chapter 6

METABOLIC MOTORS

Your body's hormonal fat burners

Diet Myths

- It's your habits that are entirely to blame for fatness.
- Your body burns most of its calories through activity.
- You can't adjust your 'slow metabolism'.

Bad genes aren't something that you wore when you were at secondary school. They're what can make you have a propensity for heart disease, baldness, mental problems and putting on weight. Though diet and physical activity play the lead roles in losing fat and maintaining a healthy weight, your genes are part of the supporting cast. It is possible to eat like a guppy but grow bigger than a beluga. Simply, some people can have a bad genetic response to a good diet (that is, they put on weight), while other people (the scoundrels!) can have a good genetic response to a bad diet.

How do we know there's a genetic component to obesity? For one, studies of twins raised apart from each other show it. Two people with the same genes raised in different lifestyles and on different diets show about 30 per cent of the same propensities for gaining weight. But genes don't just dictate how you metabolize fat – that is, whether you come from a 'big-boned' family or one that could fit through slats in air vents. Genes help dictate many things regarding why you put on fat – like cravings for certain foods or the way you cope when you're stressed. And family ties also govern whether or not the homemade sauce contains butter or olive oil.

Nevertheless, what we're trying to do is shrink the size of your jeans by shrinking the effect of your genes. While you have genetic influences that steer you towards a particular body type and behaviours, those dispositions and unhealthy decisions can be neutralized and minimized by eating the right foods, rebooting your body and, in effect, changing which of your genes are turned on and which are turned off. That's right; your choices turn on or turn off specific genes you have. For example, the flavonoids (antioxidants) in grape skins turn off the gene that makes an inflammatory protein that ages your arteries.

Now that we've discussed why you eat, how your food moves and the effects of storing excess fat, you need to know how your body burns fat. In this chapter, we'll discuss the body's natural ways of doing so – ways determined by your genes – and in the next chapter we'll discuss ways you can add horsepower to your natural fat-burning engines.

Of course, the place to start is with your metabolism, your body's thermostat – the rate at which you burn off extra fat (metabolism literally means 'change').

Most of the 1 million calories you consume every year are burned without your ever thinking anything of it. It takes energy for you to breathe and sleep, and for all of your organs to function. The energy you consume and store is used primarily to power your anatomical systems and structures.

YOU-reka!

Only 15 per cent to 30 per cent of your calories are burned through intentional physical activity such as exercise, walking or doing the wumba wumba on your anniversary. So while you may think that spinning class or Bikram yoga is the primary pathway to frying fat, physical activity is only a fraction of it. You burn most of your calories by keeping your heart pumping, your brain remembering your spouse's birthday and your liver disposing of last night's vodka concoction.

Now, that doesn't mean there aren't many outside influences that slow down and speed up your burn rate. Any movement speeds metabolism, including fidgeting (called non-exercise activity thermogenesis in scientific lingo, or NEAT for short). Every increase in body temperature of one degree increases your metabolic rate by 14 per cent (eating protein appears to do the same thing naturally, by the way). When you sleep, your metabolic rate decreases by 10 percent.

YOU-reka!

When you starve yourself for more than 12 hours, your metabolic rate actually goes down by 40 per cent. When you skip meals, your body senses a dietary disaster and quickly goes into storage mode rather than burning mode. That's the primary reason why deprivation diets don't work. Breakfast eaters are on average thinner than those who skip breakfast because they keep their metabolism genes turned on; this means that calories are more likely to be burned off before they can turn into fat.

In our battle to reduce our waistlines, we have several fearsome adversaries. And some of the greatest foes we will meet on the battlefield are our hormones. We all know that raging hormones can make a teenage boy become sex obsessed or give a menopausal woman hot flushes, but you may not know that your hormones have a lot to do with whether or not you're going to look good in a Speedo.

Is Something Secretly Making You Fat?

Before you hit yourself over the head with a stick of salami for lacking the willpower to resist aforementioned salami, or if you can't work out why you eat less than all your friends but still gain weight, consider that your hormones may be influencing your body more than you think. Glands, which make up your *endocrine system* and produce your hormones, are responsible for the genetic conditions that could be influencing your metabolism and your weight. The primary metabolic glands are:

Thyroid Gland

Thyroid hormone influences how quickly or slowly you burn energy. Too much hormone forces the body to waste energy too quickly (in extreme cases, it actually causes your heart muscle to become hypermetabolic and weaken). But if you don't produce enough, you develop a condition called hypothyroidism, in which your metabolic rate slows right down. The best way to check levels of thyroid hormone? A simple blood test. You have elevated thyroid-stimulating hormone (TSH) if it's above 5 IU/litre. This means your body is desperately trying to build up your body's circulating free thyroid hormone levels but is failing. TSH is released from your pituitary gland and tells your thyroid to produce two hormones that help control metabolism. Though decreased thyroid levels are rarely the sole cause of being overweight, abnormal levels may indicate that you should see your doctor or an endocrinologist about whether you need to supplement your thyroid function in the form of a thyroid pill to boost your metabolism. (Symptoms of hyperthy-roidism include anxiety, heart palpitations, sleeplessness and fast-growing hair and nails. For hypothyroidism, you may be lethargic, gain weight, have a reduced appetite or brittle nails.)

Adrenal glands

Adrenal glands sit like a dunce's cap on the kidneys, but they are controlled by corticotrophin-releasing hormone (CRH), which is made by the hypothalamus. This valuable relationship enables the adrenals to be very responsive to sensory input from the world around us, like a charging woolly mammoth. When chronically stressed, your adrenal glands produce cortisol, and cortisol inhibits CRH – which is too bad, because CRH will decrease your desire to eat. High cortisol levels reduce insulin sensitivity, so diabetes becomes more common and adversely influences fat and protein metabolism. The kidneys respond to high cortisol levels by retaining salt and water so that blood pressure increases. At the same time, other hormones created by the adrenal gland, including testosterone and its derivative oestrogen, increase; this can lead to obesity-linked diseases like uterine fibroids and breast cancer.

To measure cortisol levels, you need a blood test or a 24-hour urine collection. Above 100 milligrams in 24 hours generally indicates a high level of cortisol. (Note: in some people, the cutoff number varies, depending on the lab.) By the way, this is also the reason why people on steroidal medications (for asthma, for instance) seem to gain weight; cortisol is a form of steroids. (These are not

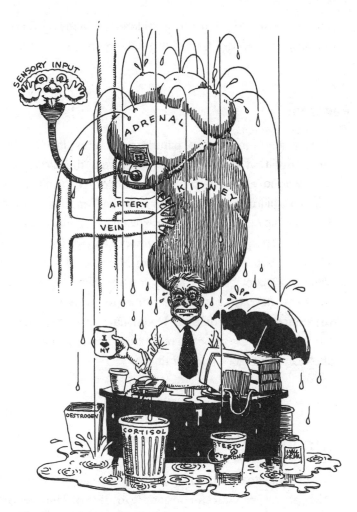

Figure 6.1 Gland Inquisition

Too much stress overstimulates the adrenal gland, which releases too much cortisol (the stress hormone), testosterone and oestrogen. This witch's brew encourages us to eat more and rapidly stores those calories in your belly fat.

the same steroids that some athletes are abusing. Those *anabolic* steroids are related to testosterone.)

Pancreas

A normally functioning pancreas secretes insulin, the substance that helps glucose travel from the blood into muscle to produce energy and fat for storage. Insulin actually works a lot like leptin; it has a mechanism that tells you to eat less. But when insulin resistance occurs in cells, it negates the appetite-control effect. Especially in early diabetes, you can naturally avoid high blood sugar with your food choices. But when you eat high-sugar foods without adequate insulin secretion to overcome insulin resistance (type 2 diabetes), you have less feedback of being full and less appetite reduction than appropriate, so the vicious hunger cycle continues.

Hormones in Action

Now, your goal shouldn't be to burn all of your fat (though you may often consider it to be so). The average person has about 2,500 calories of carbohydrate reserves – stored mostly in liver and muscle – to use for all kinds of functions that need energy, especially immediate energy, like when you're trying to catch a bus or escape a charging rhino. An average person has about 112,000 calories

FACTOID

It's not only men who get pedicures who may think they have some female hormones. All men have them – and it turns out that they're beneficial to all of us. Female hormones increase levels of HDL, whereas male hormones lower HDL cholesterol. The much higher levels of oestrogen in women may partly explain why they avoid the hardening of arteries until later in life. Many experts believe the decreased life expectancy of men is related to testosterone poisoning.

stored in fat (that is, if you are at your ideal weight, you typically have about 14 pounds of fat). The message: your body fat isn't the enemy, unless you're carrying more than you need. We need fat to function; it's an energy bank account that we can withdraw from.

The trick, of course, is to make sure we don't let our banks open up branches in every single part of our bodies.

In all, you have nine known hormones that tell you to eat more and 14 that tell you to stop eating. Hormones, like your own anatomical sports agent, are on your side. They're looking out for your health. But that doesn't mean you can't have genetic glitches. Maybe your body doesn't make leptin correctly, or your body has too much cortisol, or you can't get leptin to your brain, or none of your satiety-related hormones work at all. Those are problems no amount of willpower can overcome. Reprogramming your hormonal circuitry is the only solution. You can't beat biology, but you can make it work for you.

One perfect example of hormonal influence comes in the form of the hormone adiponectin, which we talked about in the last chapter. The more adiponectin you have, the lower your weight and body-fat percentages. (And it's directly related to omental fat, your gut fat. If you don't have omental fat, you'll have more adiponectin flying around.) It helps your muscles turn fat into energy and suppresses your appetite. Now get this: When you lose weight, *more* adiponectin is available to your body.

YOU-reka!

It's one of your body's greatest reward mechanisms. The more weight you lose, the better your body is able to deal with the inflammation we talked about in the last few chapters, because of the protective effect of adiponectin. It's one of the reasons why when you gain weight, you start increasing the irritation in your body – you produce less of this natural anti-inflammatory agent.

The Sex Factor

We all know what testosterone and oestrogen do for things like body hair, breast size and the desire to spend Saturday night rampaging between the sheets like a pair of

Graeco-Roman wrestlers. But your sex hormones can influence more than just the activity that goes on below your waist; they can also influence what happens *to* your waist.

Reproductive-hormone Friendly Fire

One of the most common causes of obesity in women comes from a condition called polycystic ovary syndrome. In fact, PCOS is responsible for 10 per cent to 20 per cent of weight problems among younger women and is often diagnosed by irregular periods and by physical appearance: abdominal obesity, acne, thinning hair and male-like hair growth (for example on the face). In the end, sufferers lose their feminine appearance.

What happens is this: women with PCOS have stingy ovaries – they get an egg all primed and ready to go in its follicle, but they won't hit send and ship the egg out. The follicle, raring to go, keeps sending out its messenger, oestrogen. Now, oestrogen works great when it gets paired up with, or balanced by, another ovarian messenger called progestin, which gets released from the egg sac (called a corpus luteum) after the follicle ships out its egg. In PCOS, some of that excess oestrogen running around gets converted to androgens, or male hormones; these cause that extra hair growth and increased appetite. That's when the pounds add on.

To combat this drive for another slice of coconut cream meringue, many women go on the birth control pill, which stops the weight gain by giving finite doses of oestrogen and progestin, telling the ovaries to quieten down. The pill alone won't cause you to lose or gain, but having less of a voracious appetite and reversing the hormonal burden of PCOS often will.

Testosterone

It may be what produces chin hair and male egos, but testosterone is also found in women and is another hormone that could play a role in weight gain in both genders. Testosterone levels tend to fall in post-menopausal women and older men; this reduces libido and can lead to weight gain because you have less muscle mass, and more calories get stored as fat. When the cause of weight gain isn't clear from other diagnoses (such as other hormonal deficiencies, including thyroid disease) and the cause of libido loss isn't clear (conflict in relation-ship, stress, vaginal atrophy), supplementation with testosterone patches or topical testosterone gels or creams could make sense not only to reverse a plummeting libido, but maybe – just maybe – to eliminate a paunch. And some argue that increased sexual satisfaction can help with satiety.

Quick note: testosterone is currently under investiga-tion and not ready for prime-time use. So before you consider treatment, be aware that testosterone has risk factors and several side effects, including acne, facial hair growth and rage reactions.

The Better Sex Diet?

There's an added benefit to healthy foods: many of them can boost sex-related hormones that increase desire – including omega-3 fatty acids and foods containing the testosterone-boosting mineral zinc. Some additional foods (think asparagus and artichoke hearts) have been linked to sexuality because of their physical resemblance to certain anatomical parts. Since it's hard to complete a double-blind randomized trial on this theme, we'll just pass along the limited facts and let your imagination do the rest.

YOU Tips!

If You Think it's Not You, Find the Cause

For some of you, it doesn't matter whether you eat like a worm or exercise like a thoroughbred; you just can't lose weight. 'Hormones' are an appropriate scapegoat for some with knee-tickling guts. If you're convinced that your fat can't be attributed to your lifestyle, it's worth asking your doctor about blood tests that measure hormone and other chemical levels to see what medications may address hormonal issues. These are the levels we'd suggest learning about:

Test	Desired Level
Thyroid-Stimulating Hormone	Less than 5 mIU/l (milli-international units per litre)
Urinary Cortisol	Less than 100 mg/day
Potassium	More than 3.5 mg
Calcium	Between 8 mg and 10 mg
Luteinizing Hormone/ Follicle-Stimulating Hormone	The individual values aren't as important as the ratio, and you'd like a 3:1 ratio of LH to FSH, no matter what time of the month.
Free Testosterone	More than 200 mg/dl for men; 20–70 mg/dl for women.

Do a Once-over

PCOS can be diagnosed with a blood test that measures total free testosterone. If your ratio of luteinizing hormone to follicle-stimulating hormone is greater than 3:1 (see above), that can also indicate PCOS. Treatment comes in the form of birth-control pills, to regulate the hormonal patterns, and the diabetes drug metformin – Glucophage – to help prevent a cross fire that happens between the ovary and the pancreas, and to calm the inflammatory responses in the liver, so that it helps the body become more sensitive to insulin.

Chapter 7

MAKE THE MOVE

How you can burn fat faster

Diet Myths

- Lifting weights will make you bulky.
- The best exercise for losing fat is cardiovascular training.
- You need weights to build muscle.

We all know that muscles give us the power to lift boxes and babies. They give us the power to walk around the shops and sprint for a train. And depending on your tastes in movie-star muscle, they have the power to make your tongue wag faster than a golden retriever's tail. But you don't have to be an appliance deliveryman or an Olympic shot-putter to benefit from muscle. When it comes to waist management, the real power of muscles lies in their ability to work like an anatomical pack of wolves. While your hormones are responsible for a large portion of your metabolism, your muscles can expedite the process of burning extra calories.

YOU-reka!

While muscles give us the metabolic ability to burn calories every time we move – during exercise, during gardening, during sex – their true advantage is that they constantly feed on calories, even when you're moving about as fast as a skateboard with a broken wheel. See, every pound of muscle burns between 40 and 120 calories a day just to sustain itself, while every pound of fat feeds on only 1 to 3 calories. Day after day, that's a huge difference in your metabolic rate and your daily calorie burn. When you add a water bottle full of muscle to your body, you're able to burn a refrigerator full of fat.

When we think about muscles, we tend to think about really big ones, but working your muscles isn't necessarily about making you big and brawny. By focusing on the right muscles and following the right plan, you won't add bulk; you'll firm up, and you'll stimulate the amount of growth needed to help burn extra calories. Best of all? You don't need any expensive equipment or a gym membership to see the benefits of adding muscle. You need only one piece of equipment: your own body. Your body is your gym.

Your Muscles: Strength Builders and Fat Burners

Your skeletal muscles – that is, the muscles attached to your bones by tendons and ligaments, not the involuntary muscles associated with working your organs, like your heart or oesophagus – come in pairs. That allows one muscle to move a bone in one direction, while the other moves it in another (when you bend your arm at the elbow, your biceps muscle pulls your upper and lower arm together, while your triceps muscle pushes them away from each other).

Now, we could bore you to a pond's worth of tears by explaining the biology of muscle, so we'll summarize what you need to know: skeletal muscle is designed to do two kinds of things – to make you fast and strong. It's made up of bundles of fibres, each of which is like a strand of spaghetti. These fibres have filaments that have to slide over each other like an expandable ladder.

When your brain sends the message for your muscles to move – to walk, to lift a sofa, to kiss your lover's ear – your muscles contract the way an extendable ladder would contract, by ratcheting the poles up and down. And it uses a catch or hook to stop the muscle and keep it opened or closed (see Figure 7.1). Now, you can build up two parts of that ladder – the actual poles, which give you strength; and the force that it takes to move those poles up and down, which gives you stamina. The force-generating structures act like calorie-guzzling cyclists pedalling furiously to pull together muscle fibres (see Figure 7.1).

FACTOID

Think of exercise as medication. Too much of a stretch? Well, studies show that exercise decreases the risk of depression as effectively as an antidepressant. Thirty minutes of daily walking has been shown to decrease the risk of breast cancer by 30 per cent and increase the rate of survival by 70 per cent. Plus, it improves the survival rates of heart attack victims by 80 per cent.

Elastic recoil generated by the contraction and aided by stretching helps the muscle relax after exercise.

The two main forms of exercise – stamina training and strength training – influence the structure of the ladder differently. Stamina training increases your muscles' capacity to produce and use the energy they need to contract, since you are adding more powerful cyclists, but muscle strength requires strength training that builds up the ladder poles – making for a bigger, stronger and sturdier muscle fibre structure. How? When you do any kind of resistance training (that is, pulling or pushing some kind of weight) you create tiny tears in your muscle fibres. Your body reacts to those tears by saying, 'If you can tear down my ladder, I'm going to build a stronger, bigger one next time.' And your body builds back bigger and stronger ladder poles. (Walking, by the way, increases both your energy capacity and your poles, which is one of the many reasons why it's a central part of this plan.) By regularly

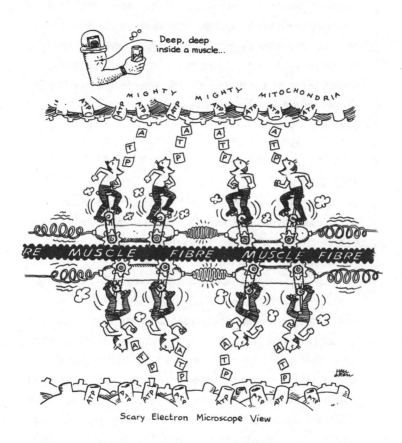

Scary Electron Microscope View

Figure 7.1 Muscle Makeup

Mitochondria create ATP from energy we consume and feed the muscle
fibres. The cells are coupled with tracks and move on one another to
shorten (lifting your body) or relax (stretching).

doing strength training, you create more muscle mass – muscle mass that you need to help you burn fat. In essence, you make the spaghetti strands a little thicker and stronger rather than making more spaghetti strands.

Muscle serves as a primary energy consumer for your body. Think of it as a raging fire. Toss a log into it, and it'll burn the log up pretty quickly. But your fat is more like one lit match – it would take years for that match to burn the log.

YOU-reka!

Add just a little more muscle, and you'll use more energy and store less fat. And that makes it an even more efficient exercise for burning fat than cardiovascular training.

That's pretty crucial when you consider that we lose an average of 5 per cent of our muscle mass every 10 years after the age of 35 – if we don't do anything about it. (Historically, hunters, gatherers and carriers of children needed their muscular strength until they were about 35, when kids were able to walk and younger tribesmen could hunt. But after they turned 35, their bodies didn't give two tubers about whether they had any muscle, so their bodies adapted and allowed for that gradual loss.) Today we see drastic effects when we lose muscle – we gain weight. If you don't intentionally rebuild muscle through exercise, every 10 years you'll need to eat 120 to 420 fewer calories each day to maintain your current weight.

So if you're at a stable weight at age 35 and don't do any kind of resistance training, while still eating the same amount of food, you'll gain weight.

Now, as your muscle ages, you also lose a little bit of the proteins that make up your muscle; they're what give your muscles the ability to have both strength and stamina. Exercise rebuilds and maintains proteins and muscle mass to prevent you from gaining weight. Here's what you need to do:

- 30 minutes of walking *a day* to help rebuild the stamina- and strength-based proteins. That prepares your muscles for ...
- 30 minutes of strength/resistance training *a week* to rebuild the strength-based proteins. (That's once a week for 30 minutes, or split up into two 15-minute sessions or three 10-minute ones.)

In Chapter 11, we'll outline the specifics of the plan, but we also want to explain that muscle is a heavyweight prize-fighter – not just in its ability to clobber fat but also because it's literally heavy. When people start to exercise and eat more healthily, their initial reaction is typically frustration, because it seems like their weight doesn't change that much at first.

YOU-reka!

That's because fat floats and muscle sinks; muscle is simply a lot heavier than fat. So as you build a little bit of muscle mass and lose fat, you may not see a dramatic reduction in scale numbers right away, but you will see reductions in waist size and overall shape. After you make it through the initial transition into exercise, chances are that you'll continue to see more dramatic changes in your body composition, your metabolism, your weight and your waist.

Now, the question is: how do we add more muscle, rather than just maintaining what we've got? And how do we do it without ending up looking like a weight-lifter?

The answer, of course, lies in exercise – but perhaps not in the way you might think. Most of us break down exercise into two categories: stamina-based training (*aerobic*, like jogging or swimming) and strength-based training (lifting weights). Any kind of exercise burns calories while you're doing the activity, but the most potent and long-lasting fat burners are created not when you're swimming or running, as you might believe, but *after* strength training. That makes muscle one of your body's greatest anatomical allies. Here we're going to show you how to take advantage of your muscles' muscle – the right way, the easy way, the way that will not only get you more stares than a Monet masterpiece but also help you get the waist that you want.

While many diet plans don't discuss the role of exercise, we consider physical activity vital to inflate your health and deflate your waist size. Building muscle is one component, but cardiovascular training and increasing your flexibility are also part of your waist-management plan. Together, the three components of exercise will have numerous effects on your body:

■ Exercise increases your metabolism so that you burn energy at a higher rate than if you didn't exercise, and it reduces your appetite by turning on your sympathetic nervous system, which activates your fight-or-flight response. Do the experiment yourself. Take a quick walk or jog when you feel the first twinge of hunger. Presto, your hunger is gone when you return.

■ Exercise will help you lose the extra weight that's stressing your joints. By dropping weight, you'll feel less pain in your knees, hips, ankles and back. And that will put you into a positive cycle of behaviour, so that you'll have the desire to exercise more.

■ Exercise stimulates the release of endorphins, which stimulate the pleasure centres in the brain. When they're stimulated, they give you a sense of control, which is associated with a decreased need to eat out of control.

■ Exercise helps decrease depression and increases positive attitude, so you make other positive choices and don't have to use food as your medication.

■ Exercise keeps your blood vessels open and clog-free, thus decreasing your risk of obesity-related morbidities like high blood pressure, elevated lousy cholesterol, memory problems and heart attacks.

We could spend dozens of pages listing all the benefits of physical activity, but we think you get the point. In fact, what's so wonderful about exercise is that unlike the things you have to take away from your life (junk foods, excuses), physical activity is something you can *add*. When you get your muscles moving in the right direction, your waist size will follow.

When you first start exercising, your body will respond with very outward signs: you'll sweat, you may feel sore, you may stink like month-old macaroni salad. Your body will also start responding on the inside, with changes in muscle size, blood flow and blood chemistry. While exercise – even combined with a healthy diet – won't suck fat out of you instantaneously, you will see and feel changes in your body shape even within a week. And with the combined

Have You Gone Too Far?

Exercising is like nuts in at least one way: there is such a thing as too much of a good thing. While exercise has more pluses than a maths textbook, you can take it too far. Burning more than 6,500 calories a week through exercise (that's roughly 13 hours) or doing more than two hours in a row of cardiovascular training not only can stress your joints (depending on the exercise), but it also appears to be the level at which you induce too much oxidative stress in your body, and that decreases your longevity.

workout and eating YOU Plan, you may see a two-inch reduction in waist size within the first two weeks as your body composition changes. So get up and get moving.

YOU Tips!

Know Your Fantastic Four

Physical activity and exercise are like vegetables; they come in all shapes, sizes and tastes, and just about all of them are good for you. Depending on your health level and experience, you need to be thinking about including these components of activity in your life:

- **Walking:** We do it at the shops, around the house, and back and forth from the fridge to the water bed. And, yes, any walking is healthy (the optimum is to hit at least 10,000 steps a day). But you also need to dedicate a total of 30 minutes a day to walking (broken up into chunks of at least 10 continuous minutes if you need to). It's the foundation for all other exercise because it not only increases your stamina but also prepares your body for strength training. As a daily routine, walking is the psychological discipline that helps you stick with an activity plan. In fact, it has the highest compliance rate of any exercise. Commit to walking, and you'll start committing to more than just the television schedule on Thursday nights.

- **Strength:** Even if the only barbell you've ever seen is the one that's piercing your friend's tongue, that doesn't mean you should shy away from resistance training. Strength training – whether you use dumbbells, machines, bands or your own body weight – helps rebuild muscle fibres and increase muscle mass, which will use up all those extra calories that you crave, so you can burn calories more efficiently and help prevent age-related weight gain. Now, here's the key to making it work: many people tend to spend a lot of time working their peripheral muscles (like their biceps or their calves), but efficient strength training comes when you work the big muscles that make up the core axis of your body – your legs, the large muscles of your upper body (like your chest, shoulders and back) and your abdominals. They're your *foundation muscles*. Best of all, you don't need a single piece of equipment to see the benefits.

  One quick note about abdominal exercises: they won't burn fat per se, but they will strengthen your entire core to help flatten and tone your stomach when you do burn fat. And they'll give you a layer of muscular support that will also protect your lower back from injury. The tighter your abs, the less excess strain you'll cause your lower back. You can't build a house from the second floor down, and, in a way, your abdominal muscles and your entire core provide a foundation that you can build upon.

- **Cardiovascular Stamina:** By doing cardiovascular exercise – that is, any activity that raises your heart rate for a sustained period of time (sorry, watching George Clooney movies doesn't count) – you'll increase your overall stamina, burn calories and improve the function and efficiency of your heart, as well as lower your blood pressure. Getting your body to sweat also helps you to release toxins that would otherwise build up in your tissues.

- **Flexibility:** Being flexible isn't just a good trait for yoga teachers and potential spouses; it's also what you want for your muscles. Good flexibility helps prevent injuries to your joints, because stretching works your muscles through a wide range of motion that you'll go through during exercise and everyday activity. Plus, being flexible just makes you feel better; it keeps your body from feeling stiffer than a week-old cockroach corpse, helps facilitate meditation and allows you to centre yourself as you focus on your body. Plus, the more pliable and loose you are, the less you're affected when you fall or get into accidents.

The YOU Diet Activity Audit

What You Need to Do	How Much You Need to Do
Walking	10,000 steps, total, accumulated throughout the day (with at least 30 minutes of continuous walking)
Muscular strength	30 minutes of resistance exercise a week
Cardiovascular stamina	80 per cent of your maximum heart rate (calculated by 220 minus your age) for 20 minutes, three times a week. For a 50-year-old, the target would be 0.8 times (220 minus 50), which equals 136 beats per minute. Also, you can measure it through exercise intensity. On a scale of one to ten, rate the intensity of your exercise. You should exercise at about a seven or eight on that scale – 70 per cent to 80 per cent of your perceived maximum.
Flexibility	Five minutes a day

Excuse-proof Your Life

When it comes to working out, most of us have two excuse cards we like to play: we have the ace of 'no time' and the jack of 'it's not convenient'. Now, we know you're busy. We know you're juggling more balls than a 12-armed clown.

We know it's easier to sit on the sofa than to do a push-up on the floor. But we also know this: time and convenience aren't excuses. First of all, with this plan, you don't need a whole lot of time (30 minutes a day to walk and 30 minutes a week to do some resistance training). If you don't have the time to do this, then you have to be willing to admit that the problem is not the fact that you're out of time but the fact that your life is so out of control that you can't budget enough time for your health and well-being.

And second, you don't need a gym or fancy equipment; it takes more time to drive to the gym and change clothes than it does to actually work out. You can do all of this activity at home – with a few modest pieces of equipment or even by making use of items you already have. In fact, in the YOU Workout, you use your body as your weights. It certainly beats spending your workout time waiting at the exercise machine for someone to finish her issue of *Quilting Quarterly*. Yes, it's easy to say you're too tired, too stressed, too busy, too this or too that. We say, too bad. The only way you'll strip away the fat is to start by stripping away the excuses.

You Move, You Lose

One unsung form of exercise: fidgeting. Studies show that fidgety people are simply skinnier people. If you have two people doing the same job and eating the same diet, the one who gets up to talk to someone down the hall rather than emailing her will be skinnier. Studies show that it isn't some mysterious food, organ, cell or gremlin that makes these people burn up fat like an iron skillet, it's these fidgeting movements. Now, that's not to say that if you go on an all-fidgeting, leg-shaking, finger-tapping programme (think Robin Williams), you'll be thinner than a Hilton sister. But numerous studies have shown that the more you move – in very subtle ways – the more calories your body will burn throughout the day. Find an excuse to move your muscles wherever you are. Clear the dishes. Stand up and walk in circles while you're on the phone. Walk down the hall to ask a colleague a question, rather then IM-ing her. Tap your toes in a meeting. Take every opportunity to move around, and you'll give your body subtle metabolism boosters that may just have more-than-subtle effects.

Squeeze Yourself

Here's an abdominal exercise you can (and should) do anywhere: suck your belly button in tight and squeeze your bum in as if you're trying to pull up a pair of too-tight jeans. Pretend the top of your head is being pulled by a string to the ceiling. Now hold that position. Besides putting you into proper posture, it's working your transverse abdominis muscle (your supportive girdle muscles). Do it in the lift, while queuing, at work and anywhere you walk.

YOU Test: How Fit Are You?

You can measure your fitness levels in different areas of activity. Use these tests to see how you stack up. (Before doing each test, make sure you properly warm up by walking or doing light exercise for at least five minutes.)

Cardiovascular: You can measure your heart's efficiency by measuring your heart rate *after* exercise. After exercising for a period of 18 minutes at 80 per cent to 85 per cent of your max (that's 220 minus your age), do three minutes at your maximum heart rate, then stop and check your pulse. Your heart rate should decrease 66 beats or more after two minutes of stopping. Do not do this without the approval of your doctor unless you do it regularly as part of your workout.

Muscular: To gauge upper-body muscular stamina, do the push-up test (men in standard form; women can do it with knees on the floor). A 30-year-old man should be able to do at least 35 (five less every decade after that, until he reaches 70). A 30-year-old woman should be able to do 45 with knees on floor (five less every decade after until she reaches 80).

Flexibility: Measure lower-back flexibility by sitting on the floor with your legs straight out in front of you and slightly spread apart. With one hand on top of the other and fingertips lined up, lean forward and reach for your feet. Women 45 and under should be able to reach two to four inches past their feet. Older women should be able to reach to the soles. Men aged 45 and under should be able to reach to the soles. Older men should be able to come within three to four inches of the soles.

PART III

THE SCIENCE OF THE MIND

How your brain chemicals and emotions
control your eating (and overeating) habits

Chapter 8

THE CHEMISTRY OF EMOTIONS

The connections between feelings and food

Diet Myths

- Hedonistic eating is triggered mainly by extreme hunger.
- Cravings are directed by taste buds.
- The best way to resist temptation is with willpower.

Our ancestors ate to survive; they ate because they were hungry or maybe to celebrate a victory over a warring tribe. Us? We eat because we're angry, bored, stressed, depressed, frustrated, watching a movie, busy, not busy enough or getting together with friends. What we think of as an emotional reaction – where we substitute chocolate for a conversation, or ice cream for a bath or crisps for a punch bag – isn't always as much about character as it is about chemistry.

Early in the book, you learned about the chemical reactions that take place in your body that stimulate hunger. Leptin and ghrelin are the joysticks that control our eating actions. But often, the physical action of eating can be triggered by emotions that coax us to wolf down the mustard-smothered hot dog. In the next two chapters, we'll discuss how the science of your brain and emotions can contribute to what and why you eat. While emotions are the least understood part of the obesity issue, they're also a very real part of overeating for many people. Your hypothalamus (remember, the site of your satiety centre) is also the part of your brain where your mind and body literally connect. As the bosom buddy of the hypothalamus, the pituitary gland sends chemicals to talk to the rest of the body. It's really where the whole weight-loss game is won and lost – this connection between physiological and psychological needs for eating.

As you well know, emotional eating isn't about reaching for celery. Rather, it's out-of-control, hedonistic eating (that often comes from your food memory), where we eat every biscuit in the packet because they look good and taste even better. It's a craving, and usually for something that's starchy, sugary, salty or loaded with fat. The following five brain chemicals are the ones that primarily influence our emotions, and not only do they provide the foundation for why we eat at certain times, but they're also the key chemicals in many of our current and future weight-loss drugs.

To deal with some of the emotions and stresses that lead to eating, you have to remember that the brain chemicals that influence our hunger and our moods are our 'why' regulators of eating.

Norepinephrine: the caveman fight-or-flight chemical. It's what tells you to tangle with a sabre-tooth or hightail it to the safety of your hut.

Serotonin: the James Brown of neurotransmitters. It makes you feel good *(Hyah!)* and is a major target of anti-depression drugs.

Dopamine: the brain's fun house. It's a pleasure-and-reward system and is particularly sensitive to addictions. It's also the one that helps you feel no pain.

GABA (gamma-aminobutyric acid): the *English Patient* of amino acids. It makes you feel like a zombie and is one of the ways that anaesthesia may work to reduce your responsiveness to the outside world.

Nitric Oxide: the meditation-like chemical. It helps calm you. This powerful neuropeptide is usually a very short-lived gas that also relaxes the blood vessels of the body.

Now, the real question is: what do all these chemicals have to do with whether or not you snack on a Twix bar or a plum? Probably the best way to think about it is to use serotonin as an example. Picture your brain as a small pinball machine. You have millions of neurotransmitters that are sending messages to and from one another. When your serotonin transmitters fire the signals (from the flip-pers), they send the message throughout your brain that you feel good; this message is strongest when that feel-

Mood Foods

Recent research shows what many of us knew all along: our moods dictate what we eat. Researchers studied the diets of people to show how personality and foods collide – how our moods may steer us to certain foods, on the basis of their physical characteristics. The study theorized that many moods send specific signals; for example, stressed adrenal glands could be sending salt-craving signals. So what does your favourite turn-to food say about you?

If You Reach For ...	You May Be Feeling ...
Tough foods, like meat, or hard and crunchy foods	Angry
Sugars	Depressed
Soft and sweet foods, like ice cream	Anxious
Salty foods	Stressed
Bulky, fill-you-up foods, like crackers and pasta	Lonely, sexually frustrated
Anything and everything	Jealous

good pinball is frenetically bouncing around in your brain. But when you lose the ball down the chute (that is, when cells in the brain take the serotonin and break it down), that love-the-world feeling you've just been experiencing is lost. So what does your brain want to do? Put another coin in the machine and get another ball. For many of us, the next ball comes in the form of foods that naturally (and quickly) make us feel good, to counteract the drop in serotonin that we're feeling.

Unfortunately, the way we typically satisfy our urge to play another ball is to use the foods that provide an immediate rush of serotonin. That rush can come with a jolt of sugar: sugar stimulates the release of serotonin. Insulin facilitates serotonin production in the brain, which in turn boosts our mood, makes us feel better, or masks the stress, pain, boredom, anger or frustration that we may be feeling. But serotonin is only one ball in play. You have all of these other chemicals fighting to send your appetite and cravings from bumper to bumper.

To see how the total picture works, think of these chemicals as parts of a scale. When the chemicals associated with positive feelings (like serotonin or dopamine) are in the up (or activated) position, you're chemically high. But when they're down, you experience a big chemical downfall (see Figure 8.1).

YOU-reka!

And this puts you in a state of anxiety that sends you searching for the foods, especially those simple carbohydrates, that get you back to the chemical high. That's how illegal drugs work too; users keep seeking the high not always for its own sake but to avoid the lows. You're constantly fighting to get back to that place of neurochemical comfort. When these chemicals are high, your weight gets lower, and when they're lower, you reach for the foods that eventually make your weight higher.

That's the reason why what happens under your skull plays such a vital role in what happens under your belt. Knowing how your emotions can steer your desire to eat will help you to resist your cravings and, ideally, avoid them altogether. Your goal: keep your feel-good hormones level so that you're in a steady state of satisfaction and never experience huge hormonal highs and lows that make you search for good-for-your-brain-but-bad-for-your-waist foods. In the next chapter, we'll explore this further – with the deeper emotions that can contribute to eating, hunger and weight gain.

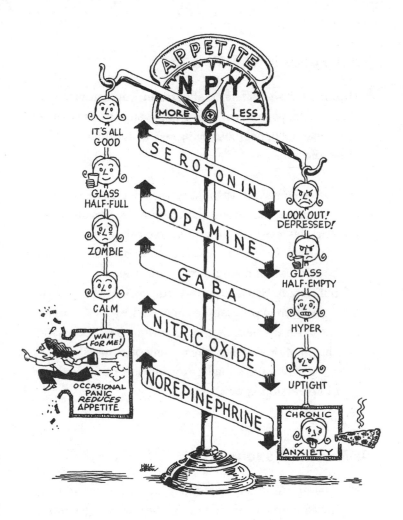

Figure 8.1 Scale of Injustice

Brain hormones that control emotions also influence appetite. Not having enough of each pulls the scale towards more NPY – and more appetite.

YOU Tips!

Work Foods in Your Favour

Foods all have different effects on your stomach, your blood and your brain. These are some of the nutrients that may influence your hunger and the brain chemicals that affect it:

- Turkey contains tryptophan, which increases serotonin to improve your mood and combat depression, and help you resist cravings for simple carbs.
- Omega-3 fatty acids, which are found in fish, have long been known as brain boosters and cholesterol clearers, but they've also been shown convincingly to help with depression in pregnant women. Depression, as we'll explain in the next chapter, contributes to hedonistic and emotional eating. Since many of us have low omega-3 intake, it might explain some other instances of depression as well.

Savour the Flavour

If you're going to eat something that's bad for you, enjoy it, savour it, roll it around your mouth. We suggest taking a piece of dark 70 per cent cocoa chocolate and meditating – as a healthy stress reliever and as a way to reward yourself with something sweet. We're trying to find small ways to make you feel good and increase serotonin, so you don't plummet and scavenge for anything you can find. It's okay to eat bad foods – every once in a while. It's not the first piece that's going to do the damage; it's scoffing the whole bag that will.

Go to Sleep

Getting enough sleep keeps you thin. That's because when your body doesn't get the seven to eight hours of sleep it needs every night to get rejuvenated, it needs to find ways to compensate for neurons not secreting the normal amounts of serotonin or dopamine. The way it typically does that is by craving sugary foods that will give you an immediate release of serotonin and dopamine. The lack of sleep throws out your entire system – even increasing your levels of NPY, which increase your appetite. Lack of sleep can become an even bigger factor as you age. When you get older, the pineal gland in your brain produces less of the sleep hormone melatonin, resulting in a craving for carbohydrates.

Chapter 9

SHAME ON WHO?

The psychology of the failed diet

Diet Myths

- The diet would work if only you had the willpower of a lean person.
- It's better to have dieted and failed than to not have dieted at all.
- You can't make mistakes when you're dieting.

Most diets aren't about action; they're about thoughts. By their very nature, they force us to think, think, think, think. Diets make us think about food more than inmates think about escape. You have to think about calories, or zones, or the hour when you're next allowed to have half a cracker. You think about not having food so much that you develop only two sets of standards when it comes to eating: either you follow your diet or you don't. It's bean sprouts or it's prime steak. It's carrots or it's biscuits. It's cucumbers or it's pepperoni. It's all or nothing.

In a way, we've all been thinking too much about weight and what to eat, and not enough about how and why we eat. When most of us try to lose weight, we pull out the most powerful weapon we'd like to think we know – our brains – and launch a psychological attack in the form of discipline ('I can resist this food!') and ego ('I'm smart enough to avoid this food!'). But as you'll see in this chapter, the truth is that there are very strong emotional triggers that make us eat – and make most diets fail. In many ways, it's our brains that sabotage our best dieting efforts.

By trying the very thing that's designed to help us lose weight – a diet – we've created a no-win system of failure that spins us into a cycle of blame. And what's not to blame? The experts blame our societal fatness on cheap junk food. Or we blame our fatness on magazine covers (for the unrealistic body images that taunt us to smear our self-esteem in daily fistfuls of cheesecake), 60-hour working weeks (for making us sit down all day), cloud-soft recliners and reality television (for making us sit down all night), and so on.

But deep down in your gut (there, over by the sticky buns you ate two weeks ago), there's really only one thing you blame for the size of your gut:

You.

You blame *you.*

You tell yourself it's not the restaurants or food manufacturers or deep-fried cheese-stuffed peppers that are derailing your weight-loss efforts, it's your mind. The entire battle of the broken belt comes down to a flurry of mental 'if onlys' – and your perceived inability to control what food you shuttle down your oesophagus year after year, day after day, meal after meal, bite after bite. If only you had the willpower to step away from the mayonnaise. If only you could stop after four Pringles. If only you had the power, the strength, the discipline, the chutzpah, the energy, the drive and the motivation to control your waist, then you'd *finally* have the body you want.

What you're really doing here is laying brain blame. We rely on our minds to resist temptations, to make smart decisions, to eat right, to know better and to make healthy choices. So we naturally rely on our minds to combat the emotions that we think we should be able to handle – stress, anxiety, depression (studies show that those with higher levels of all these emotions are more likely to be overweight or obese). So when we give up on a diet and balloon to a size that makes doorways cringe, then we automatically think something's wrong with us, that our minds aren't strong enough to win over our waists.

The reason we fail? Researchers theorize that it's your mind that might be crossed up, but not because of anything you're doing. At least scientifically, overeating may work a little bit like drug addiction; in fact, studies show that obese people even have reward centres in the brain similar to those of drug addicts.

So let's say you're stressed. Remember the hypothalamus and the chemicals that change according to your moods. At points of stress, you've activated neurotransmitters from a part of the brain called the locus coeruleus. Your body, in response, tries to calm those neurotransmitters and combat the stress. Some people do it with cigarettes, some do it with food, some do it with sex, some do it with drugs. When you combat the stress with food, you're also activating the reward centre of your brain. And then, after that initial feel-good system wears off, you'll reach again for the same thing that made you feel good, calm and relaxed: food. That's why stress and anxiety make it that more difficult, neurochemically, to stick to whatever plan you're trying to follow.

What's especially interesting is that right next to the hypothalamus, where the feeding and satiety chemicals

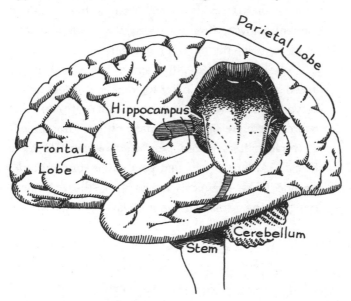

Figure 9.1 Food for Thoughts

When you eat sugar, you light up the motor cortex of your brain, which controls your lips, tongue and mouth. The hippocampus, which controls memories of food, lights up when people on rigid diets crave certain foods – overwhelming their willpower and ability to resist.

NPY and CART are produced, is a part of the brain called the mammillary body (because it physically looks like a pair of breasts). That's where food memory is stored, so when you get the signal that you're hungry, you're also accessing your memory of and cravings for foods you've eaten in the past – which may have been bad foods. Plus, the parietal region of the brain – the control centre of the movement of the tongue, lips and mouth – acts differently in heavy people than in skinny people. Brain scans show that in heavy people tempted with sugar, this region becomes activated. In skinny people the region stays dormant, showing how sugar can play a role in emotional eating for some people but not others.

If you've struggled with waist issues, you've probably placed all the responsibility for dietary success or failure on your little three-pound brain. But you can't outwit nature. There are simply too many of those hormones and neurotransmitters whose jobs roughly translate to 'pass the cake'. And to expect that your *will* or your *fortitude* can override these chemicals messages is the equivalent of trying to stop a train with your pinkie.

Dieting: Avoiding the Issue

For a second, think about one particular kind of person – the extreme example of fat gone wild. These people are often the stereotypical ideal – funny, kind, generous, charming, articulate, creative and more brilliant than a perfect diamond – except for the fact that they're regularly mistaken for a four-story silo. (We all say it: 'He'd be so great, if only he were *thin*.') And that bothers us. It bothers us that we can't work out the yin and yang of the situation. How can a person smart and driven enough to have a successful career be the very same person who, night after night, gets clobbered silly by a helpless packet of chocolate biscuits hiding in the back of the cupboard?

Something has to be wrong.

And it is. The issues aren't at waistband level; they're at brain level. You may know you have health problems and a waist circumference the size of Neptune. And you may even know that you struggle with the emotional issues of confidence and esteem that come as the side dishes with the main course of obesity.

YOU-reka!

But you may not know that you could be what's called an avoider, in that you suffer internally from a tornado of psychological turmoil that comes with the public and private disdain for obesity, and you avoid confronting your situation at all because of the internal fear of not being able to beat it.

Here's how avoiders think (nod if this sounds familiar): once you deviate – even slightly – from a diet or healthy eating plan, you think that you might as well drop the whole thing. (Nodding?) And this starts a cycle that avoiders can't find a way out of: we're fat, we try to lose weight, we deviate just a little, we fear rejection for the perceived failure, we isolate ourselves from people, we stop talking about it, we stop the diet, we mow through a pound of cheesecake, we get fat. And then we try to lose weight, and the cycle continues.

Avoiders at all levels (from the extreme cases to the milder ones) will see their weight bob up and down like a bull rider. Physiologically, it's a never-ending cycle of weight gain and loss (that's called weight cycling). But the real avoider issues stem from the psychological effects of weight cycling. Instead of avoiding bad foods, avoiders tend to want to avoid other things – like the people who want to help them and the discipline of trying to eat healthily. Above all, avoiders try to separate themselves from these two strong emotions associated with dieting.

Guilt: 'I Hope They Don't Find Out'

No matter what kind of diet you may have tried in the past, you've undoubtedly worked with a list of off-limits foods. High-protein diets might ban potatoes. Low-fat diets might ban cheese. Sugar-busting diets may ban you from ever setting foot in Aunt Thelma's kitchen again. Inevitably, like a child instructed not to touch the champagne flutes, you will want potatoes, you will want cheese, and you will find it incredibly rude to turn down Aunt Thelma's lemon meringue pie three times in a row. So you cave. But because you've set yourself up with a list of banned foods, you perceive half a biscuit, or a hunk of Gouda, or three measly fries as first-degree diet homicide: the diet's dead. And that's where guilt sets in – from the fact that you know you deviated from a predetermined set of standards. That holds true for all levels of avoiders. We all identify with nutrition-induced guilt, and then we make a subconscious decision that it's easier to deal with the effects of being overweight than it is to feel the boulder-heavy guilt every time we want to smother a carrot in blue cheese.

Shame: 'Oh Gosh, They Did Find Out'

For the person who feels they cheated on that diet – whether it was a simple kiss with a Kit Kat or an adulterous romp with a vat of ice cream – there's an even worse feeling than guilt. And that's the shame associated with dietary infidelity. You've cheated, so you now feel you lack the strength to succeed. So what are you going to tell your spouse and all your colleagues who've been watching you feast on iceberg lettuce at lunch for the past eight days? That, yes, you're a failure? You could last on your diet for only a week? You have one little thing you're doing, and by gosh, you can't even keep a stinking croissant out of your mouth? The public humiliation, or just the perceived threat of possible embarrassment, primarily stems from that societal disdain for obesity. This shame – a much more profound emotion than guilt – spins you back into the cycle of avoidance: It's better to not be on a diet and be fat, the avoider calculates, than to be on a diet and eventually prove to the world that you can't succeed.

Research shows it's better for your health not to diet at all than to say you're dieting and steal spoonfuls of crème brûlée during every commercial break. That's because diets typically promote weight cycling and yo-yo dieting (gaining and losing, gaining and losing), which are actually more hazardous to your health than keeping a steady overweight weight. (That's probably because most weight cyclers eventually gain more than they lost and suffer the slings of shame.)

Avoidance is a normal thought process: when you reach an obstacle, you decide that instead of trying to find a way around it, you might as well turn around and go back to the beginning. One of the strategies for handling emotional eating is to live and eat in the present – not being upset about what you ate in the past and not obsessing about what you'll eat in the future.

Why Our Brains Aren't Equipped for 'Dieting'

Unfortunately, the very thing that's designed to help people lose weight is the very thing that promotes this behavioural and psychological pattern: diets that promote the all-or-nothing mentality.

It turns out that much of the diet dogma we've all accepted as fact is more hype than horse sense. Like a tantalizing trailer that creates expectations well beyond what the film can deliver, the problem with most diets is not with the preview; it's with the plot. The typical diet drama opens to reveal the hero dieter preparing for battle – attacking the enemy head-on. Armed with grit, determination and little else, the hero prepares for battle against flying chocolate sundaes in a quest for total domination over food. But what our hero doesn't realize is that the secret weapon she was counting on will never arrive; the cavalry is nowhere in sight. So the battle becomes gruelling, mentally and physically exhausting, and never-ending, and all this hard work tends to create quite an appetite, and the energy halo from yesterday's feast of three sticks of celery and a cherry tomato is quickly fading. Our hero needs a pizza, and fast.

YOU-reka!

If you make one small move like this, research shows that you'll be three times more likely to follow through with the specific plan you intend to follow. This small change is your way of putting the key in your waist-management ignition (www.mychoicescount.com can help).

Unfortunately, much of the dieting mind-set comes from the initial expectation we set. When you're ready to go on a diet, you set the rules, you know the parameters, you know that veggies are nutritional heroes and biscuits are

Can You Spare Some Change?

We all know that making a change in your life is as mental as it is behavioural. Research shows that this is the best four-step process for making change:

Be Positive. It works for coaches, bosses and parents, as well as waist managers. If you blame yourself for your weight, if you are depressed about your weight, if your mood is fouler than an underground station in August, then your first job is to refocus. You need to think about what you can do, how you can do it, why it's good for you and how you'll succeed. In the weight-loss game, poker-faced confidence trumps negativity every time. By stripping yourself of the negative emotions of guilt and shame, you'll make the right rational (and long-term) decisions about your eating obstacles.

Add Some Support. You may not know it, but your world is full of saboteurs – people out to make you fatter than Microsoft's coffers. There's the boss who brings in sweets every Thursday meeting. The friend who brings you a pie when you're upset. The spouse who suggests pitchers of margaritas and a plate of cheese nachos to celebrate the end of the week. Maybe there's nothing wrong with their intentions, but there is something wrong with the fact that their attempts to appeal to your heart are actually damaging it. What we want you to do – no, *need*

nutritional mass murderers. That process and anticipation of going on a diet can work in your favour, as long as you remember that the way your brain works isn't just psychological but chemical as well. Many diets leave you less wiggle room than one of Beyoncé's dresses, so that there you to do – is develop a support system of people who know your goals, know your obstacles, know your weaknesses and know your strengths. (Don't have anyone? You can hook up on the Internet, including on www.realage.co.uk.) This person will be your sounding board, your comfort system and your measure of accountability. With public accountability – that is, you reporting in on those daily struggles and successes – you're more likely to make a permanent change.

Make a Gesture. Just making a seemingly small change will help determine your long-term success, whether it's buying a pedometer, a health-club membership or new walking shoes; throwing away the unhealthy foods in your cupboards; and even setting up a computer file to record your progress.

Then Do It. Once you start with the small gesture, you're ready. Eat a full day's worth of perfect-for-you food. Walk for 30 minutes today, tomorrow and every day after that. That's right, 30 minutes of walking a day is the minimum commitment. (You can break it up into smaller segments if you can't do it all at once.) Then make a second action commitment: commit to doubling (or tripling) your daily vegetable intake. With one foot, take one specific first step. The next foot has no choice but to follow.

are only two options: rewards for compliance and no toler-ance for failure.

In just about every other area of our lives, we allow ourselves margins of error. Lawyers don't win every case. Parents don't always make the right decisions. In fact, almost all of us make mistakes in our daily jobs. We learn from them and try to correct them so we don't repeat them again and again, or at least work out how to minimize the damage. But when it comes to diets, we hold ourselves to the precision of a Red Arrows flight team. No errors. No mistakes. Once we've blown it and deviated even an inch from our plan, that's it. Diet's dead. Pass the fondue pot.

Through the tips below, you can learn to reprogram your mind to strip away the guilt that comes with eating, the guilt that comes with diets, and the guilt that comes with occasionally enjoying foods that aren't at the platinum level of healthy-eating charts. You also have to realize that it's not the first chip or slice of cake that will doom your diet. It's the second, the third and the whole shebang that lead to dangerous fat and waist gain.

At the beginning of our plan, you do have to listen to your body and respond intelligently to your cravings and your emotions. But over time, you'll learn how to eat right and manage your cravings. And that's when you'll train your brain to stop obsessing about eating right – and punishing yourself for every obstacle you face.

YOU-reka!
The unrecognized truth is that when you stop overthinking, you'll stop overeating.

The Role of Soul

The reality is that a good number of us with weight problems have emotional issues that run deeper than the middle of the Pacific, and we try to satisfy our need for a higher power by self-medicating with food.

If you're one of those people, you don't much care about leptin, ghrelin and NP-whatever.

Being overweight is more about self-esteem – about the petrifying fear that you don't *deserve* to be thin. How do we know this? Not through studies or research – but through real-life living, through our patients, through eavesdropping on a cavalcade of doughnut addicts. Here, we have to step out of the safety zone of hard science into an area that's typically not studied by the white-coat-and-goggles set, because the mental, emotional and deep psychological issues involved with obesity are simply very difficult to 'prove' in a Western sense.

So let's start here: many people – women especially – lack the self-esteem for waist control. (In fact, the most common reason a woman doesn't take care of her own health is because she puts others' needs before her own.) But let's dive deeper: what *is* self-esteem? Let us assume our general sense of self-worth comes from two forces: overcoming obstacles and accomplishing some kind of goal. In the case of waist management, what happens if you don't overcome an obstacle (the box of chocolates) and don't accomplish something (your goal weight by your school reunion)? Yes, your self-esteem plummets faster than ratings for summer reruns. To resurrect it, you need to find ways to overcome and accomplish – without making the very standards by which you measure your life unrealistic weights, measurements and stricter-than-boot-camp eating habits.

Now, let's step back to see how the relationship developed between the emotional need for self-esteem and the physical need for baggy clothes. In our youth, many of us long for something in our lives that's deeper and greater than our everyday reality of work, home, sleep, repeat for 29,930 days. Maybe it's religion or a calling to help others. We don't care as much *what* the 'It' is as that we *find* the 'It' and *explore* the 'It'.

Now, there are some chemical and biological foundations for that feeling of soul-level satisfaction. Oxytocin, a hormone that is elevated in women after childbirth, also makes you feel a sense of community and pleasure within your family, or during a religious experience, or when you have an epiphany about your existence. When levels of oxytocin increase, you feel calm. Another hypothesis argues that your sense of self-esteem and well-being is influenced by the chemical nitric oxide (not to be confused with the laughing gas nitrous oxide). Traits such as hopefulness and optimism are associated with the release of nitric oxide through the body. In the same way, the release of nitric oxide may serve to help reduce feelings of anxiety and stress. But this chemical effect lasts for only seconds, so you need to continually stimulate your body with the right cerebral karma.

Soul-level satisfaction exists at a biochemical level as well as in your perceptible life. It's your deeper drive – not the drive to fill the needs of your stomach or your muscles or even your mind, but the drive to fill the needs of your soul.

Okay, we know what you're saying: what does your soul have to do with the fact that you just scoffed an entire can of whipped cream?

A lot.

For many of you, instead of addressing – or even acknowledging – this deeper longing and the restlessness you feel for never quite fulfilling it, you try to fill the emptiness with food and drink. You use a temporary fix to satisfy the permanent void caused by not satisfying your spiritual needs (the 'It').

Sound familiar? We bet it does. Of all the actions you pursue, one of the few things you totally control is eating. You have the freedom to eat what you want, where you want, how you want, and whether or not you want to do it with or without clothes on. Because of that freedom, eating makes you feel good. Funny thing, though; food is like the paint you use to cover cracks formed in the foundation of your house. Two coats of robin's-egg blue may hide the flaws temporarily, but they're never going to fix the real root of the problem.

YOU-reka!

If this is you, your cover-up is what starts that tornado-like cycle that keeps you from ever feeling satisfied physically or emotionally. Ask yourself: could this be part of a cycle?

- You long for something deeper ...
- And when you can't find it, you eat to feel better ...
- But you feel lousy because you gain weight ...
- Then you tell yourself you don't deserve to be thin because you can't keep weight off ...
- Then your self-esteem drops further because you haven't overcome obstacles or accomplished what you want ...
- So you self-medicate with food ...
- And then you medicate yourself with food when you can't find 'It' ...

What's especially interesting is that many people who use food as a cover-up *want* to live life in the tornado. They're terrified by the thought of being thin. Being fat gives them an excuse to fail, an excuse to be depressed, an excuse to tango with a Twix bar.

So what does the theory say about why many people do this to their own bodies? Or *why* you'd do it to your body? You may do it because this thought process is a safe one and because your fat serves as a literal and metaphorical protective layer that keeps you from inter-acting with reality. You don't have to play the game of life if you're constantly making excuses for living on the bench. If only you could lose weight, if only you could fit into that bikini, if only you could take a hike with the family without breathing more heavily than an escaped prisoner. While some people may say that fat is a failure, the truth is that fat – for many of us – is a way of avoiding failure, because it's an excuse for never competing and engaging in life.

So where do you go from here, short of self-injecting oxytocin or inhaling high doses of nitric oxide? It's not like you can turn this page and all of your self-esteem issues will vanish. It will take some time, but it also takes some awareness that this tornado may be swirling. We're not asking – or expecting – you to fix it. Simply realizing that you may use food as a psychological painkiller is part of the solution for helping you avoid it. So let's just consider that the warranty on this emotional baggage has run out. Now that you know this baggage doesn't serve you, it's time you dropped it off at a psychological landfill and got rid of it for good.

YOU Tips!

Make the Split

Clearly, some of us eat for physical reasons (we're just hungry) and some of us gnaw on leftover Halloween sweets for emotional reasons (we're annoyed at the boss about having to start and finish a new report by 10 a.m., and it's 9:47). But sometimes it's not always easy to work out the difference. To help, you need to start using the YOU Diet Hunger Test. Throughout the day, record your level of hunger as judged by this scale. Stay tuned to what your stomach is telling you, not what's happening outside with stresses (kids going crazy), emotions (spouse is working late *again*), or habits (*Coronation Street* equals two chocolate biscuits). This process will help you really *feel* your hunger, so that you can let your stomach, not your emotions, dictate your habits.

O Tank = Hungry. It feels as if you haven't eaten since the first year of secondary school.

1/2 Tank = Edge is off. You're okay, not desperate, like maybe when you're driving home from work.

3/4 Tank = Satisfied and not hungry. You can go much longer without food. You just ate nuts and had a drink before dinner.

1 Full Tank = Full and comfortable. It's the way you feel after finishing an average-portion, healthy meal.

Overflow Level S = Stuffed. You could've stopped two scoops of pudding ago.

Overflow Level OS = Overstuffed. Audible groaning detected.

Overflow Level BP = Button Pop/Exploding. It's the typical Christmas Day gorge. You feel sick, and even take the name of your mum's stuffing in vain.

Every time you find yourself reaching for the cheese sauce or biscuit tin, rate your hunger. Then think about whether you're reaching for the leftover lasagne because you're truly hungry or for a reason that has absolutely nothing to do with hunger. Ideally, you'll want to stay in the ¾ to Full Tank range – satisfied at all times. And you'll get there by eating regularly throughout the day. (See Part IV for details.) After applying these gauges for two weeks, you'll start to instinctively know why you're eating, and, better, you'll train yourself to eat simply to keep your stomach satisfied – and not your emotions.

Pick and Stick

Yes, variety may be the spice of life, but it also can be the death of dieting. When you have a lot of choices for a meal, it's a lot easier to slip out of good eating habits. One way to get away from fat bombs is to eliminate choices for at least one meal a day. Pick the one meal you rush through most and automate it. For most people, it's lunch. So find a healthy lunch you like – salad with grilled chicken and olive oil, turkey on wholegrain bread – and have it for lunch every day. Every day. Yes, every day.

YOU-reka!

More and more research is showing that putting a cap on the variety of foods and tastes you experience will help you control your weight. How does it work? It seems that when you have meals rich in flavour variety, it takes more and more calories to keep you full. So when we experience meals with lots of diverse flavours – think Mexican or Indian cuisine – we tend to eat more to satisfy our taste buds. Now, we don't want you to become bored with food, but if you make this a habit for at least one meal a day, it'll decrease your temptations and help you stop thinking about food so often. In fact, we usually prescribe two meals that are the same each day for our patients. Another trick: use extra-light virgin olive oil, which has less flavour and may help control taste cravings.

Find a Substitute

How can you take irrational, emotional and addictive actions and turn them into smart, rational good decisions? For one thing you can develop that list of healthy contingency foods and clear your fridge and cupboards of waist-killing foods, which we'll show you how to do in Part IV. For another, you can look for other things to fill the needs that food is currently filling. Traditionally, so much of our self-satisfaction comes from how we see ourselves externally. But that satisfaction is fleeting, and we need to find and focus on the things in life we're truly grateful for – be it our families, our careers or a hobby that we're passionate about.

Keep Your Hands Full

You'd think that being plopped in front of the television playing Xbox would mean that you're destined for a life of fatness. But that's not the case; studies show that playing video games is actually not correlated with obesity. Why? Turns out that when you've got your two hands on the controllers and your fingers moving faster than Liberace's, that means one thing: your paws won't be in a packet of crisps. (Some games even have foot mats for you to make commands with your feet, too, so you can get a complete workout; ask your kids about the Dance Dance Revolution craze.) Now, that's not to say that an intimate relationship with Super Mario should be your number-one strategy, but it does prove an underlying point.

YOU-reka!
When you keep your hands and brain occupied –
whether it's with video games, gardening or
removing a spleen – it means you're putting your
brain in the state you want: not thinking about
eating and not automatically reaching for something
to put in your mouth.

Walk This Way

The root of the YOU physical activity plan is a minimum of
30 minutes of walking a day (broken up into three
segments of 10 minutes each if you need to) – and telling
somebody about it after you're done (yes, every day, no
excuses). You will do it not only for the physical effects,
but also (even more so, actually) for the psychological
effects. Remember what self-esteem comes from: the ability to overcome obstacles and achieve goals. Walking
accomplishes both.

Get Lost in Your Mind

Whenever you feel the urge to eat, just sit and think about
your life and what's driving you to pick up a fork or open
the fridge. Would you shove that stuff in a friend's or family
member's body? It's okay to cry, to think, to meditate.

In fact, maybe you can learn from your pain – not make it worse by thinking you can pad it with three extra inches of abdominal fat. For some, meditation or prayer enhances their power to satisfy the subconscious drive they have.

Get Touched

Both on a physical level and on a psychological level, seek out positive interactions with other people. (Remember the phone call at the end of your walk.) Evidence shows that increased amounts of oxytocin may be able to decrease blood pressure and lower the effects of stress. And the way research shows that you increase oxytocin levels is through CCK, which helps control your appetite, and through an increase in social interaction and touch. If nothing else, it's a good reason to schedule that weekly massage. And it may help reinforce why things such as meditation and hypnosis – suspected to increase oxytocin – can be helpful with weight loss. Also, while there's as much information on this as on obesity in elite marathon runners, the fear of touch and lack of oxytocin release may be one reason why the abused individual often has problems with waist management.

YOU Test: Why Ask Why?

The fact is, you *know*. You know if you need to lose weight. You can tell by the way you look, by the way you feel, and by whether your clothes feel tighter than an unopened pickle jar. But to be able to make changes – sustainable changes – you not only have to know *what* you've done to your figure. You also have to know *why* you're abusing your body, in the form of the emotional and physical triggers that led you to gaining waist. To start, perform a self-administered 'why' test – that is, keep asking yourself 'why' questions about your weight until you come to the real answer about why you want to lose weight and why you can't. It may go something like this:

Why do you want to lose weight? Because I want to fit into my old pair of jeans.

Why do you want to fit into your old pair of jeans? Because I'd have more confidence.

Why do you want more confidence? Because I'll feel better trying to meet new people.

Why do you want to meet new people? Because I'm recently divorced and hoping to start a new relationship.

Why do you want to start a new relationship? Because I'm feeling lonely …

And that's likely to be where the thread of questions stops – where you can link the first question to the last answer. You want to lose weight because you're lonely, but the likely cause of your weight gain is the very same thing: that you're lonely.

YOU Test: The Personality Test

Take this personality test to see what attitudes and behaviours may be preventing you from losing weight and getting healthy (Dr Robert Kusher's full test is available at www.diet.com). Add up your ticks and see how your attitude towards eating and exercise influences the size of your waist.

EATING PATTERNS

Sounds Like You?	Tick	Because It Means You're a ...
'Day to day, I change my meal patterns often.'		**Meal Skipper:** You skip meals and have no pattern or routine to when you eat.
'I eat like a sardine during the day and like a humpback at night.'		**Night-time Nibbler:** You consume 50 per cent or more of your calories between dinner and bedtime.
'The place I'm most likely to eat: one that has a waiter, a drive-through lane or a delivery service.'		**Convenient Diner:** You're a brand-name eater. All of your meals are packaged, bagged, microwavable or frozen.
'Fruits and vegetables have the same taste appeal as, oh, sewage.'		**Fruitless Feaster:** With few exceptions, you're all about meat and potatoes (or pasta, bread and desserts).

Sounds Like You?	Tick	Because It Means You're a ...
'I need a dietary restraining order. If there's any food within 50 feet of me, I'll eat it.'		**Steady Snacker:** Besides your regular three meals, you snack anytime you come near food.
'I pile my plate as high as I can.'		**Hearty Portioner:** You eat a lot, and you eat it quickly, whether it's healthy or not.
'I eat salads when I'm out with friends, then raid the cupboards when I'm home.'		**Swing Eater:** You eat a strict diet of good foods, but fall off the wagon and then overeat bad foods.

EXERCISE PATTERNS

Sounds Like You?	Tick	Because It Means You're a ...
'I enjoy being physically active as much as I do making paper-clip chains.'		**Couch Champion:** You don't like to sweat, and you don't really like any physical activity.
'I don't exercise because everyone else at the gym looks like a supermodel or Schwarzenegger compared to me.'		**Uneasy Participant:** You hate exercising in public because of your body image.

Sounds Like You?	Tick	Because It Means You're a ...
'I like exercise, but if I have to miss it, it's hard for me to get back on track.'		**All-or-nothing Doer:** You work out hard for a few days or weeks, then stop and do nothing for even longer.
'For the past three years, I've been doing the exact same workout without changing it a bit.'		**Set-routine Repeater:** You're on a fixed exercise routine but aren't able to lose weight because your body has adjusted to the routine.
'I'm afraid I'll get hurt on the wrong end of the exercise machine, worsen my condition or have a heart attack if I exercise hard.'		**Tender Bender:** You either have an injury that prevents you from exercising or worry that you may suffer one because you're out of shape.
'I'd like to exercise, but I barely have enough time to shave, let alone step on a treadmill for 20 minutes.'		**Rain-check Athlete:** You're so busy and frustrated that you can't make time to exercise.

COPING PATTERNS

Sounds Like You?	Tick	Because It Means You're a ...
'Ahhh! I find food as comforting as a down pillow.'		**Emotional Eater:** You eat when you're stressed, anxious, tired or depressed.

Sounds Like You?	Tick	Because It Means You're a ...
'As for my clothes, I've got a bigger cover-up plan than a criminal – I'm ashamed of my body and how I look.'		**Self-scrutinizer:** You feel ashamed of your body and have trouble separating body image from self-esteem, and that affects your day-to-day decision making.
'I'm the Socrates of diets – I spend more time thinking about what I need to do to lose weight than actually doing it.'		**Persistent Procrastinator:** You know the importance of losing weight and say you want to lose, but you never seem to make it happen because something always gets in the way.
'I'm juggling more than a circus performer. Last on my list? Time for myself.'		**People Pleaser:** You are a good-natured person with responsibility and commitment to family, friends and colleagues, but you always put them ahead of you.
'My life is moving fast, my to-do list is the length of a novel, and I can't find the brakes.'		**Fast Pacer:** You multitask and don't take the time to think or plan how to improve your lifestyle.
'I've tried everything to lose weight, but nothing ever works. Nothing!'		**Doubtful Dieter:** You say you've tried everything and nothing works, so you develop a self-defeating attitude.

Sounds Like You?	Tick	Because It Means You're a ...
'My work? Great. Family life? A blast. I expect the same amazing results from my weight-loss plan – but my progress is never enough.'		**Overreaching Achiever:** You're successful at home and work – and expect the same in your weight loss. But you never feel satisfied, and your high expectations make you feel frustrated and discouraged.

Adapted from *Dr Kushner's Personality Type Diet*
(St. Martin's Press) with permission.

Check Yourself: Add up your scores and get a score for food (eating), mood (coping) and movement (exercise). The dimension with the highest score is the category where you need to focus. A score of four or more in any one category means you need to focus on that area no matter what. So, if your food score is six, mood score is four and movement score is two, then you need to focus on food and mood, but don't forget your 30-minute daily walk – no excuses.

YOU Test: Don't Avoid This Test

It shouldn't come as much of a surprise that avoiders typically have feelings of inadequacy and are hypersensitive to being negatively evaluated. Identifying with four or more of the following statements means you have strong avoidance tendencies.

- I avoid work activities that involve close interpersonal contact – not because of my deodorant level but because I fear criticism or rejection.
- Unless I know I'm going to be liked, I'm hesitant to get involved in relationships.
- When I'm in social situations, I feel more inept than an umpire with a detached retina.
- My shirt's not coming off unless the lights are going off.
- All of my social situations feel like school; I'm preoccupied with being criticized or rejected.
- I don't engage in risky activities because my biggest fear is the risk of embarrassment.
- In new interpersonal situations, I feel the same way I feel at the beach: shy and inhibited, and I would do anything to be somewhere else.

PART IV

THE YOU DIET AND ACTIVITY PLAN

The eating and activity plan that will become lifelong and automatic

Chapter 10

MAKE A YOU-TURN

How to change what you thought you knew
about dieting – and change your life for good

By now, you don't have to be Marie Curie to know the power of chemicals and realize that you're the clear-cut underdog if you try to take them on with brute force. You know that chemical changes in your brain and body play a big role in dictating everything from your actions to your emotions. But you can alter your chemistry in more subtle ways. For instance, take the act of positive thinking and interacting in social groups. There's evidence that those kinds of actions change serotonin levels to make you feel better and reduce appetite. That's really how you should be using your mind and all the intangible concepts like willpower, discipline and motivation – to complement the chemical changes you're making in other, more concrete ways. They're the things that will help you overcome the occasional butter-laced obstacles that you'll face.

To show how you can use emotions to work for you as you're about to embark on the YOU Diet, let's step back into the mind of a typical dieter – let's say a woman. One of the psychological realities of being overweight is that many dieters – that is, people who know they need to lose weight and want to – are somewhat comfortable with their bodies. Yes, that body may be 20, 30, 40 or more pounds heavier than it was the day she turned 18. But maybe she's used to post-pregnancy weight, she enjoys Friday lunches with her friends, or she can't face a total wardrobe overhaul.

YOU-reka!

It's who she is – and she's more comfortable living her life at that level than going through the struggles and hard work (not to mention the guilt and shame) of trying to shed weight.

So the dieter has two choices: she can remain on top of the hill where she's currently standing and (relatively) comfortable. Or she can try to get to the top of that beautiful mountain in the distance – the ultimate destination for all of her weight-loss goals. There, on the mountain, she'll find smaller sizes, fewer doctor visits and probably fewer health risks and an improved quality of life. Maybe that's where she'd *ideally* like to be. But the problem is that there's no easy bridge from the comfort zone of the hill to the peak of the mountain. To get there, she must travel all the way down from her current comfort level, hit some rough terrain along the way, and then climb, climb, climb her way up this seemingly insurmountable incline. So she asks: is it worth going through all the hard

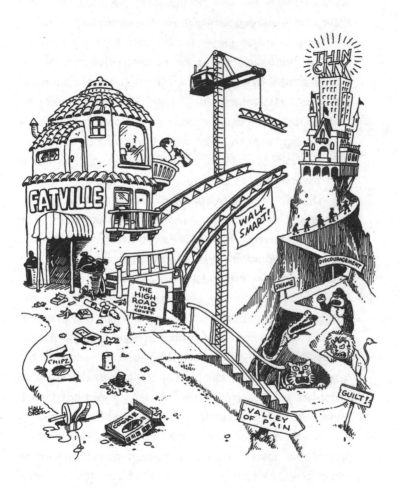

Figure 10.1 The Right Route

Descending into the valley can make the trip up to the promised land daunting. Dieting smartly will build you the bridge you need to transition to your playing weight.

work to reach the top of the ideal mountain, or am I comfortable enough with where I'm standing right now?

That's how the dieter thinks after trying it once or twice. It's easier to stay at the current comfort level at a less than ideal size than it is go through a short period of somewhat uncomfortable change – doing things like developing a physical activity programme, or avoiding drive-throughs, or changing menus, or going through periods of irritability and hunger. For many dieters, that path is hard to navigate, so they return – very quickly – to the original hill, the original place of comfort (often it is an even wider hill, psychologically and waist-size-wise). The fact is, most people aren't willing to face the challenges of finding the mountain peak, even if the peak reveals such vistas as better health and higher self-esteem.

So what we have to do is build that bridge – that bridge of smart food choices, of exercise discipline, or working smart, not hard. And we have to support the bridge with strategies and tactics that allow you to make wrong steps without falling completely into the abyss of chocolate nougat. How do we do it? By getting started. Right now. With small actions that lead to big changes.

Sometimes, we think the motivation to start a programme has to come first, but often, the motivation comes after the action: make a small change (be it walking 30 minutes a day or eating nuts before dinner to keep you full), and suddenly you feel motivated to make more changes – and to succeed.

The point is that we want you to make it across the bridge as pain-free as possible, by giving you the tools to avoid the uncomfortable feelings associated with dieting, with hunger, with evil scales. The journey to the top of the mountain may feel like a little bit of a climb, but it shouldn't feel like you're starting way down there at the bottom. We'll build that bridge with these strategies and our YOU Diet and YOU Activity Plan.

YOU Tips!

Adopt the YOU-Turn Mantra

If you've ever ridden in a car with a GPS satellite navigation system, you know how it works. Plug in your destination, and the system – using satellites to plot your current and final points – tells you exactly what to do when. Turn left after 400 feet. Stay straight. Get in right lane. But let's say you make a mistake and miss a turn or turn onto the wrong street. The GPS doesn't berate you, doesn't scold you, doesn't tell you that you might as well drive off a cliff. Instead, all it says, very politely, is this: 'At the next available moment, make an authorized U-turn.' The GPS recognizes the mistake matter-of-factly and simply guides you back onto the right road. The GPS allows for mistakes and tries to help you correct them.

That's the kind of mentality we want you to have. You're going to make wrong turns. You're going to turn left at the hamburgers, make a right at the cheesecake and occasionally merge onto the motorway of fish and chips. Does that mean you should steer off the dietary cliff and fall into the fatty crevasse of destructive eating? Of course not. What it means is that you need to pay closer attention to the road signs and the instructions about how to make it to your final destination. It also means that you can't beat yourself up with a basket of croissants every time you lick a little whipped cream off your finger. So what you're going to do – right now – is acknowledge that you will face obstacles. And instead of falling into the avoidant and defeatist mentality by drop-kicking healthy eating the moment you make one bad choice, you will confront it. How? By repeating the YOU Diet Mantra:

'At the next available moment, make an authorized YOU-Turn.'

'At the next available moment, make an authorized YOU-Turn.'

'At the next available moment, make an authorized YOU-Turn.'

Get back on the right road.

What kills any regimen of healthy eating isn't the occasional dessert or slice of pizza; it's the cascade of behaviour that happens after the initial indulgence. Use this mantra to steer yourself back. Why does it work?

- It gives you a mental crutch to carry when you're faced with difficult eating situations.
- It reminds you to be confident, to be positive, to know that the harm isn't in the first mistake; it's in not working out how to deal with it.

- It reinforces the grand scheme of this whole plan – the reason why you're trying to manage your waist. The long-term benefits to your health far outweigh what you're giving up in your Pyrex dish.

Know Your Fighting Weight

In all likelihood, the way you've measured your so-called dietary success or failure is by pounds lost. If you've lost down to your target weight, then you've won. If not, you've lost. But the reality is that over the long term, all of us will intermittently gain and lose small amounts of weight, even when we're trying to lose it. For one, our water weight often fluctuates depending on what we're eating. The reason why so many low-carb dieters lose weight fast is because the lack of carbohydrates causes them to lose glycogen stores from their muscles, and with this loss of glycogen comes a loss of a lot of water; as soon as they reinstate the carbs, the glycogen comes back to the muscles and attracts the water. That adds the pounds right back. So the first five to eleven pounds of weight loss on a low-carb diet is the fake loss due to a temporary loss of water.

Instead of tracking your weight by a single goal weight of, say, 145 pounds, what you're going to do is pick your weight class. You're going to pick a range of weight that's comfortable for you – say, 142 to 148 pounds (or 31 inches to 33 inches of waist size). When you divulge your weight to someone (not that anyone will be asking), it should never be in one number; you need to think of your weight as an ideal range. For one thing, this allows for the natural fluctuations that occur. For another, it does something even more crucial to your psychological success: it stops you from focusing on some arbitrary number that promotes the idea of all-or-nothing success or failure. And it puts your mind in the right programming mode – to remind yourself that your body is supposed to change.

Stay Accountable

You can use your weight range to tell when you're pushing the upper boundaries of your ideal weight/waist with periodic checks using a measurement tool – be it a tape measure around your waist or a scale. Whatever your accountability tool, we suggest checking it every Saturday around midday to keep yourself honest with your weight and waist class. Think of your body as a rubber band. Stretch it a little, and it can certainly snap back into shape. But once you stretch it too much, it's going to lose its shape and make it more difficult – if not impossible – to return to the original size.

Plan to Fail – and Develop Contingency Plans for When You Do

We keep tyres in our boots in case one goes flat. We keep candles in our drawers in case there's a power cut. We keep backups of files in case our computers crash. And that's good; contingency plans give you the mental assurance that you'll be able to adapt to unexpected crises. But the one area where we don't make backup plans is in our diets. We eat broccoli, fish and fruit for three days, then splurge on a double-fat burger with supersize fries on the fourth. For so many of us, that's grounds for euthanizing the diet right away – putting us right back in touch with our three favourite food groups of chocolate, crisps and biscuits.

Instead, start carrying a dietary contingency plan – a diet emergency pack for those times when you may experience a crash-causing blowout in one of your meals. Follow this three-step contingency plan to help you cope with occasional mishaps and potential catastrophes. Exercise it the moment you feel you're deviating from your waist-management plan:

- **Mental:** Say the YOU-Turn mantra 10 times. Let the mantra remind you that it's okay to stray occasionally, that you can take control of the situation and steer yourself back, and that the positive reinforcement and confidence that come with overcoming challenges will give you the mental strength of a tank. Plus, the relaxing aspect of it will help influence your serotonin levels in your favour. And it will help distract you, which is what you need when you're making a beeline for the bonbons.
- **Physical:** Do a yoga pose or try the hippie stretch (see the YOU Workout). We suggest the downward dog pose, balancing your weight on your hands and feet with your bum hiked towards the ceiling in an inverted

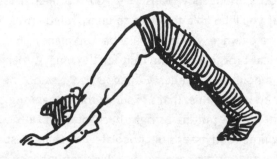

V. Not only will it help you refocus, give you a few
moments to take deep breaths and remind you of your
goals, but it will also work because it's sort of difficult
to eat when you're upside down.

■ **Nutritional:** Keep in your fridge a container of baby
carrots, celery or any crisp vegetable of your choice, or
a favourite apple type (yes, types matter to our
individual taste choices). Carrots and apples are perfect
anti-stress foods because, one, they have just a tinge of
sweetness to satisfy that craving, and, two, they give
you something to crunch into at times when you really
want to sink your teeth into your boss's neck. This will
become your turn-to food – that is, the food you turn
to when you feel angry, frustrated, mad, sad or upset –
as well as the one that will help you feel better about
the nutritional mistakes you may have just made.

Many of us take the mental approach that the only
way to 'do a diet' is to do it perfectly. But that's setting
us up for failure and shame, because it never works.
Success comes with persistence – persistence to
overcome challenges, persistence to see the big picture,

persistence to work hard enough in the beginning of the plan so that good habits become automatic.

Make it Automatic

Think of your waist-management plan a little like the way you'd drive to work. Maybe the first day in a new job in a new city, you took the motorway. But then you found out it was more clogged than Rapunzel's shower drain. So you experimented with a few back roads, shortcuts and bypasses until you found the very best way to get to work. Now you don't need a map; you do it automatically, and you don't spend a single nanosecond worrying about what turn you take. It's automatic – just the way your approach to eating should be. When you're starting out on this plan, you'll experiment with different routes, get stuck in a few traffic jams, maybe even get a little lost along the way. But if you stick with it and find the right course, you'll automate your habits, regulate your chemicals, and make eating the easiest trip you've ever made.

How do we make it automatic? By using the tools that we've outlined in the book.

Chapter 11

THE YOU ACTIVITY PLAN

Physical strategies for waist management

The world has all kinds of gyms: home gyms, hotel gyms, female-friendly gyms, muscle-head gyms and gyms that look like spas. Though any of them may be perfectly decent places to pump your muscles, work your heart or admire spandex, there's one gym that gives you absolutely everything you need:

Your own body. Your body can be your best gym.

Really, all you need are two things: your body and the knowledge of how to use it. No barbells, no dumbbells, no balls, no ankle weights, no machines – just your body. By learning and using a plan that requires only your physiological barbells, you have all the tools you need to make exercise easy and automatic. That's because:

- Your body costs nothing to use.
- You eliminate the best excuses for avoiding exercise, like driving hassles or needing to buy equipment.
- Using only your body, you can work all of the muscles necessary for effective waist management – and that's for both beginning and advanced exercisers.

In fact, you can complete an entire workout that hits all three areas of activity – strength, flexibility and cardiovascular –in one easy 20-minute workout three times a week (or do it in smaller bits for almost as much benefit). And you can change that workout no matter what your skill level, simply by making small exercise adjustments to perfectly match your abilities.

Whether you're a newbie to exercise or an old pro, the YOU plan starts with walking for 30 minutes a day – no matter what. Only when you've mastered that, no matter how long it takes, should you begin the rest of this programme.

The YOU Activity Plan

Every Day:

- **Walk:** Walk for 30 minutes. No matter what. No excuses. It doesn't matter if you do this in one whole block or broken up into as many as three shorter sessions.
- **Stretch:** Once your body is warm (after walking, for instance), stretch for five minutes to help elongate your muscles. You'll find stretches detailed in the You Workout below and the yoga poses we've outlined later.

Three Times a Week:

Do the 20-Minute YOU Workout. Do the exercises in this order; in general, you'll strengthen a muscle and then stretch it. If you want to break the workout up into smaller sessions, pick and choose as you like, but always try to match the strength and stretch exercises for a particular body part – that is, work your legs with a strength exercise, then do the stretch exercise immediately after it. Also, on the other four days of the week, you can simply take all the stretches outlined below and turn them into the three- to five-minute post-walk total-body stretch.

The 20-Minute YOU Workout

Do the following movements in order. Make adjustments to time or repetitions as your ability level dictates. Each strength exercise is followed by a stretch to loosen the same muscle group and keep you limber. On non-workout days, you can just do the stretches (labelled with an S) after walking for a short flexibility session. See www.realage.co.uk for video of each move.

How to Exercise the Right Way

1. Look out at eye level or above to spare your neck and keep you from rolling your shoulders forwards.

2. Assume the Botox pose: keep your face relaxed and tension-free.

3. Relax your shoulders and lift up your chest.

4. Pretend the top of your head is being pulled up by a string to elongate your spine and keep you from rolling forwards.

5. Count your reps of each exercise out loud; this counting will help you remember to breathe continuously and keep you from holding your breath.

6. Keep your abs tight and pulled in to support your lower back. (Practise sucking in every time you enter a car, bus, train, plane, lift, escalator – that way it becomes automatic.)

7. Keep your knees slightly bent, so you don't lock them.

8. When doing shoulder exercises, make sure you could always see your hands (if you wanted to).

9. Breathe. Many people hold their breath while doing strength training.

10. Keep moving in between exercises to keep your heart rate fast, or move directly to the next exercise. If you're unable to hold a conversation, you're exercising too hard. If you can keep a conversation going and are able to fill the listener in on all the details, you may not be going hard enough.

11. As you get stronger, go longer rather than harder with cardio exercises, and stronger with weight exercises. That is, do more repetitions of any non-weight-bearing exercise. That will help prevent injuries from overexertion. If you really feel weak, just hold the exercise position without moving and slowly work up. It's more important to follow perfect form and do fewer repetitions than to do a lot of repetitions with form that's sloppier than spaghetti in a high chair.

1: Roll with it

Allows any kinks in your shoulders to be smoothed out
Roll your shoulders forwards for a count of 10 and back for 10. 'Swim' shoulders back for 10 and forwards for 10. Your goal is to get full range of movement with your shoulders. Notice any areas that you don't move fluidly and try to open them up by relaxing as you move your hands in full circles. Between sets, get into the habit of rolling your shoulders five times forwards and five times back.

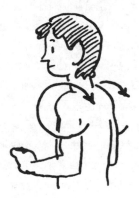

2: The Chest Cross

Strengthens chest and shoulders
(A) Reach your arms as forward as possible at shoulder height, and twirl your hands back and forth like you have a tennis ball in your hands. (B) Then, cross your straight arms in front of your chest in a series of quick horizontal motions with your palms facing each other (so they provide some wind resistance to your motion). (C) Next

move your hands rapidly up and down with your palms facing the floor. Try to do each of these variations 25 times.

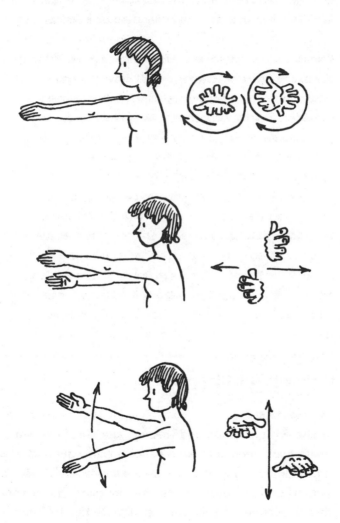

Preparation for Perspiration

Before beginning an exercise programme, you need more than a Lycra top. Exercise isn't dangerous, but your risk of injury will be less if you follow a few principles to protect your muscles and your entire body.

Warm Up. Before beginning any exercise, warm up your muscles for about five minutes to prevent injury. (The YOU 20-minute workout includes a warm-up, but if you're doing another activity, follow these guidelines.) Remember, your muscles are like spaghetti strands; they're pliable when they're warm, and more injury-prone if they're not. Jogging, brisk walking, cycling or doing exercises with light weight or no weight will help prepare your muscles for activity. One good rule: do the same exercise you will be doing but at a slower pace or with lighter weight. Your goal is to move your joints through the same range of motion as they will do with exercise — to raise your heart rate and to increase the temperature of your muscles, which will make them more viscous and less likely to be injured. Some advocate that at the end of exercise, you should cool down with a light jog, cycle or walk, but there's no evidence that a cooldown will reduce injury or muscle soreness more than just stretching at the end. But if you are doing intense cardio exercise, you do

3 (Stretch): The Clapper

Stretches chest

In a standing position and keeping your chest up, clap in front of you; then bring your hands behind your back and clap your hands together. Keep your hands as high as you can in front and back during the movement. Keep your chest lifted when clapping at the back. Do this 10 times.

need to do a cooldown, rather than stopping abruptly at the end of the workout. For a cooldown, do the same activity, like running, at a much slower pace than you were maintaining during your workout.

Focus on Your Muscles. Take special notice of where you tense up. You want to release tension in your body, not shift it somewhere else. Most commonly, people shift it to their shoulders and their foreheads. Notice this, breathe, and focus on the muscles you are working.

Listen to Your Body. Throughout stretching, make sure to keep breathing freely and slowly. If you ever feel pain during stretching, stop. (That's different from a little discomfort as you're loosening up; actual pain should be your warning to stop. We *want* burning in the muscles.)

Wear the Right Shoes. You'll need to invest in a good pair of lightweight running shoes for walking (the strength workout you should do barefoot). They're well cushioned and designed to handle the heel-to-toe movements for both walking and running. Best option: go to a sports shop, where the often underpaid salespeople are the experts; ask the pro there to analyse your stride and match up the best shoe for your feet.

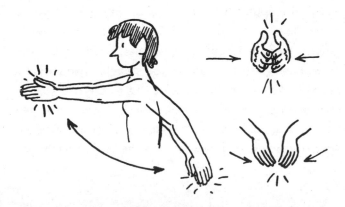

4 (Stretch): The Hippie

Stretches hips and hamstrings
With your feet flat on the ground, bend forwards at your
waist. Alternate bending one knee and keeping the other
leg straight (but still keeping your feet flat), and let your
head dangle down, releasing all your tension. Stretch each
side for 15 seconds.

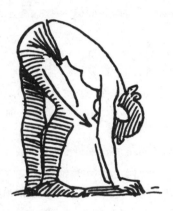

5: Push-up Pride

Strengthens chest
Get in the appropriate 'up' push-up position for you by
either staying on your toes or keeping your knees on the
ground. Lower yourself until your chest nearly touches the
ground and push back up. As you straighten your elbows,
push your spine towards the ceiling to exercise (to help
engage your back muscles as well). Pull your heels away
from your shoulders, keeping a long, solid body. Don't let
your stomach hang down towards the ground; make your

stomach active by pulling it in to support your lower back. This will help release any unnecessary tension on your lower back. Keeping your stomach tight in any exercise strengthens your belly muscles. If your lower back starts to hurt, raise your bum slightly and curl your tailbone by tightening your bum. Keep your chin slightly up and look six inches past your fingertips. This forces you to use your chest and not overextend your neck while doing push-ups. Do as many push-ups as you can (this is called exercising

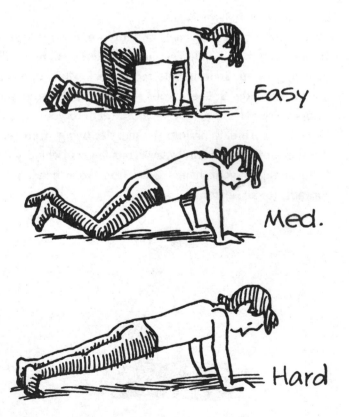

Easy

Med.

Hard

to failure, and it's what helps build strength proteins in your muscle). If these are too hard, just hold your chest off the ground without moving. Or you can do a pyramid push-up routine: do five push-ups, then hold in the up position for five seconds. Then do four and hold for four in the up position, all the way down to one.

6 (Stretch): Pecs Flex

Stretches chest and arms
Sit up straight on your heels and interweave your fingers behind your bum, while keeping your arms straight. Lift your fingers up, knuckle side facing back, while opening your chest wide. Squeeze your shoulder blades together to open your chest more. Use your breath to your advantage here, by breathing into the muscles being stretched. Another option is to interweave your fingers behind your head and pull your hands away from your head. Face forwards for all versions.

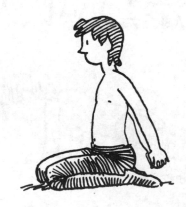

> **FACTOID**
>
> **In any ab exercise, pull your stomach muscles in. If you push your stomach out, then that is how your muscles will form. Relax your face and don't furrow your brow. This can also help avoid a future plastic surgery consultation.**

7: Steady on the Plank

Strengthens abs and shoulders

Get into a push-up position with your elbows and toes on the floor, while pushing the area between your shoulders towards the ceiling and keeping your stomach pulled in towards your lower back, to support it. Keep your buttocks tight and your eyes looking at the floor (ignore the fact that you suddenly realize you have to vacuum). Hold the position for as long as you can. If you can last more than one minute, make it more difficult by dropping your chin 20 times out in front of interweaved hands, or by trying to balance on one foot.

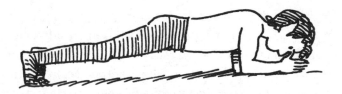

8: Whose Side Are You On, Anyway?

Strengthens obliques (the muscles at the side of your abdominals)
Turn to the side by putting an elbow on the floor and rotating the opposite hip towards the ceiling. Keep your body in a straight line and resist pushing your bum back. Keep your abs tight as you hold the position for as long as you can. Alternate sides. If you can hold for more than one minute, you can increase the difficulty by repeatedly dropping your hip, tapping it on the mat, and bringing it back into the lateral plank.

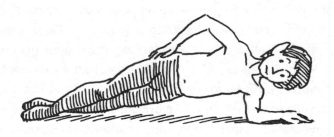

9 (Stretch): Up, Dog, Up

Stretches abdominals and obliques
From a down push-up position, with your hands below your shoulders, lift your chest and torso up into the air so that your upper body is nearly perpendicular to the floor as you come onto the tops of your bare feet. Lean

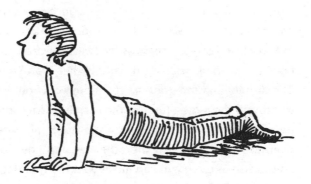

backwards to stretch your abdominals, but keep your bum relaxed. Hold for 10 seconds. Then look over your right shoulder for 10, then your left shoulder for 10, then back to centre.

10: The Rickety Table

Strengthens upper back and bum
Put your hands and knees flat on the floor with your fingers spread apart and pointing directly forwards. Keep your back flat and parallel to the floor and your supporting

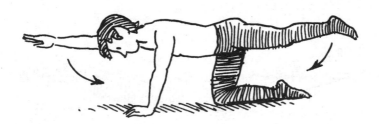

elbow slightly bent. Look down six inches above your fingertips. Reach your right hand forwards and your left foot back and stretch them as far away from each other as possible, keeping your right hand higher than your head. The higher your arm goes up, the more work your back has to do, and the more effective the exercise. Now bring your right elbow to your left knee. Do 20 on this side, then alternate and do it with the other leg and arm. For more advanced exercises you can move your arm and leg out at a right angle from your body, keeping them above your spine, and hold them there for 20 seconds. Your stomach should be pulled in the entire time, supporting your lower back.

11: Superman

Strengthens lower back
Lie flat on your stomach, reaching your arms out in front of you with the palms down. Spread your extremities straight out in all four directions and lift your arms and legs simultaneously for enough repetitions to cause some mild fatigue. Continue to look down during the movement,

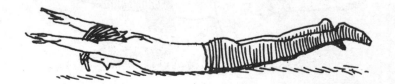

and don't overextend your neck up. This exercise is about how long you can make your body stretch – not how high you can get it. Focus on squeezing your bum as you lift. Try to make it to one minute.

12 (Stretch): The Seated Pretzel

Stretches lower-middle upper back and hip

Sit down with your legs stretched in front of you. Bring your right foot up and set it down on the outside of your left knee. For back support, put your right hand behind your right bum cheek. Bring your left toe straight up. Reach your left hand up as if indicating 'stop' and drop your chin. Then twist to the right and bring your left triceps to the outside of the right thigh. To go deeper, twist more to apply pressure against your right thigh. Act like a string is pulling the top of your head up to elongate the spine. Breathe by expanding your rib cage like you are blowing up a balloon. Really concentrate on taking deep breaths every time.

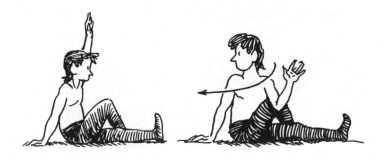

Note for exercises 13 and 14: for all reclining abdominal exercises, keep your lower back flat on the ground. Pretend a coin is trapped between the floor and your lower back, and keep your belly taut to train your stomach to be flat. As soon as you feel your lower back tenting up, stop and pull it back down as flat as possible before continuing. If this gets too hard, stop and hold it down as flat as possible for 30 seconds. Pretend there is a dumbbell tied to a string attached to your belly button, and it is pulling your stomach down towards the coin.

13: Leg Drop

Strengthens entire abdominal area
Lie on your back with your hands on your chest and put your knees at a 90-degree angle and your feet in the air. Drop your heels down, tap the mat, and bring back up to 90 degrees. Do as many as you can (to failure). As soon as your lower back starts to arch up, return to 90 degrees; keep pushing yourself a little bit further each time with your back glued to the coin. Beginners, do one leg at a time. Advanced, do it with straight legs.

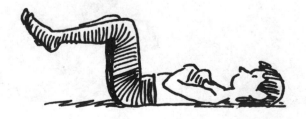

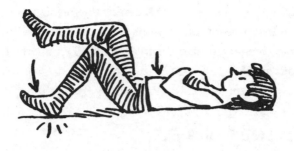

14: X Crunch

Strengthens upper abdominals

Lie on your back with your feet on the ground and your knees at a 45-degree angle. Cross your arms behind your head, putting your opposite hand to the opposite shoulder to form an X behind your head. Rest your head in this X and keep your neck loose (in the beginning, you can put a tennis ball under your chin as a reminder). Using your abdominal muscles, crunch up about 30 degrees from the floor. Without holding your breath, you need to suck in your belly button to the floor to tighten the natural girdle you have (it's a muscle called the transverse abdominis) to keep the entire six-pack tight. Also pull up your pelvic muscles (like when you are holding in your pee) to

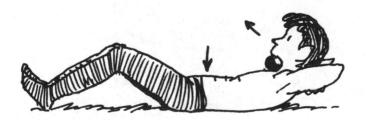

strengthen the bottom of the natural girdle. Do as many as you can, looking up towards the ceiling the entire time. Then repeat Up, Dog, Up (exercise 9) to stretch your abdominals.

15: Seated Drop Kick

Strengthens quadriceps

Sit with your legs straight out in front of you. Bend your right leg up with the knee pointing towards the ceiling. To keep your back straight, interweave your hands around this knee. Act like there is a string pulling from the top of your head, elongating your spine (and don't bob your head). Lift your straight left leg six inches off the ground, keeping your left toe pointed towards the ceiling. Lift 25 times, then switch legs. Do each leg twice. The only body part that moves is the leg; for variation, lift leg and move side to side.

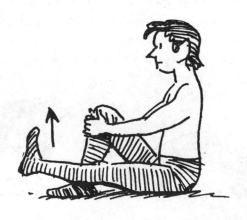

> **FACTOID**
> You can add a balancing element to almost any exercise by tweaking it slightly. Try doing two-legged exercises on one leg, or do an exercise lying on a stability ball instead of a bench.

16: Invisible Chair

Strengthens entire leg

Sit in a chair position (with no chair!) with your back against a wall, and with your palms resting on your knees. Ideally, have a stool below you, so you can grab it or sit on it when you're done. Keep your heels directly below your knees and at a 90-degree angle; your relaxed shoulders should be rolled back and the back of your head should be against the wall. Hold for as long as you can, and try to work up to two minutes. Keep your face relaxed and breathe.

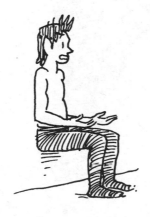

17 (Stretch): Nice Thighs

Stretches quadriceps

While standing on one leg, bend the knee of the opposite leg and grab the foot behind your back with interweaved fingers (or use one arm to hold something to keep balanced). Pull the foot towards your bum while lifting your chest forwards and squeezing your shoulder blades together. Keep your knees together. Switch legs. Keep your abs pulled in the entire time, to support your lower back. Hold each for 20 seconds.

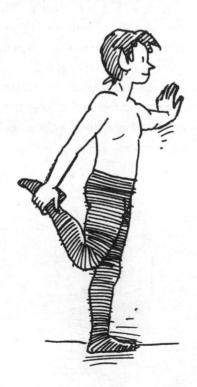

Are You Well Equipped?

Hooked on sweat? Then consider these add-ons to your physiological gym.

As You Get Stronger: Weights	Great Addition to a Home Gym: Exercise Ball
Though you can use household objects for resistance exercises, it can be worth investing in a pair or two of dumbbells to use for lunges, squats and other exercises as you get stronger.	Once you establish a fitness foundation, these large, inflatable balls are wonderful to use for crunches and any other exercise in which you sit on the bench or floor. They help you develop balance and work your stabilizing muscles in your abdominal section. They are also great stretching devices. See www.realage.co.uk for examples.
For the Traveller: **Bands**	**For Balance and Agility:** **Skipping Rope**
Resistance bands allow you to increase resistance as you get stronger, and they're also small so you can take them as you travel.	They're cheap, and easy to use. While raising your heart rate, they'll also test and improve your agility.

For At-Home Cardio: Rebounder	Versatile Bonus: Weighted Vest
Once you progress to doing cardio exercise, you can jog, swim, row, cycle or do whatever you like to get your heart pumping. If you're one of our highly coordinated readers, one of the easiest ways to work your heart is with either a skipping rope or a mini-trampoline called a rebounder. You know about the skipping rope, but for a rebounder, you can store it under your bed, pull it out and do mini joint-safe cardio sessions by hopping and jumping on it for the allotted time. (Take a quick lesson before using it, so you can learn the safety rules.)	This vest carries extra weight to give you resistance (many are adjustable so you can change the weights in one-pound increments), and you can use it for all of the central exercises, like lunges, squats, crunches and push-ups.

Cardiovascular Workout

In a week, you need 60 minutes of an activity that raises your heart rate to 80 per cent of maximum (220 minus your calendar age). You can choose from such activities as running, cycling, swimming, rowing or using an elliptical trainer. (Vigorous sex also counts, but here it has to be continuous minutes, so it's unlikely this'll be a good alternative.) For the last one to four minutes, raise the intensity to the highest level you can for the maximum benefits. Then cool down for five to ten minutes on low intensity of the same exercise. If you do the YOU Workout, above, at a level that raises your heart rate, these 20 minutes of sweating can count towards your weekly cardiovascular exercise total of 60 minutes a week.

Note: When doing exercises with your own body weight feels too easy, you can add resistance by holding dumbbells or plastic bottles filled with pebbles, sand or water, or using other household products, like soup tins.

Chapter 12

THE YOU DIET

The waist-management eating plan

Whether or not you're the kind of person who skips the plot to get to the ending, you've arrived. Welcome to the YOU Diet – our reprogramming plan provides you with the tools to make smart choices and with the strategies that allow you to make YOU-Turns after you've made bad choices.

With this plan, you can expect to lose up to two inches of your waist size within two weeks. As you launch into this 14-day rebooting program (it's actually so easy that it's one seven-day plan done twice, so you can do it perfectly

---

Fill 'Er Up

About 20 minutes before dinner, eat ½ ounce of walnuts with 1 cup of your favourite YOU Soup. Or drink at least 8 ounces of water with 1 tablespoon of psyllium. Either will help fill you up so you won't want or need to eat as much to feel satisfied.

A Portion of the Plan

Many experts will tell you that the key to successful dieting comes from two words: *portion control*. That makes sense, but not in the way you might think. We emphasize that you eat healthy portions of food (about a fistful per serving) and use nine-inch plates not to restrict your calories per se but to slow you down. If you can slow your calorie intake, you'll give your brain a chance to keep up – and activate the right amounts of leptin and ghrelin to keep you satisfied. So, start with the right servings of food, take your time eating them, then gauge your levels of satiety (using our fullness gauge on pages 192–3). If you're still hungry, then have another serving (the size of a fist, not the size of a head) of a good-for-you food.

and learn to do it automatically), remember this: your body is made up of hundreds of beautiful biochemical instruments, and they all play different notes, melodies, harmonies and chords within your anatomical orchestra. As the conductor, you direct how those notes are played and what kind of sound they'll make. Like any new piece of music, the YOU Diet will take a week or two for you to learn it, for you to feel it, for YOU to become ingrained. But once all this happens, your orchestra will play like never before.

The YOU Diet Crib Sheet

Meal Strategy	Three main meals plus snacks, so you're never hungry. No eating within three hours of bedtime. Consider dessert an every-other-day treat.
Waist Foods (Eat 'em)	Whole-grain carbohydrates; fibre; nuts, which include healthy monounsaturated and polyunsaturated fats; protein such as lean meats (two-legged preferred) and fish.
Waste Foods (Trash 'em)	Added sugars, simple carbohydrates, fructose as in high-fructose corn syrup, trans fat, saturated fat, non-whole-grain flour and enriched and/or bleached flour.
In a Hunger Emergency	Apples, almonds, walnuts, edamame (soya beans), sugar-free gum, water, cut-up veggies, low-fat yogurt and cottage cheese, or pre-made YOU soup.
Substitution Foods	In any recipe or meal plan, you can replace any fruit or vegetable with another to make recipes to your taste.
Meal Journal	You can keep track of what you eat at www.mychoicescount.com.

Supplements	Once a day, take a multivitamin as an insurance policy against less-than-perfect food choices. (It's even better if you split the pill and take half twice a day.) Through food and the multivitamin, you need to get a total of 1,200 milligrams of calcium, 600 IU of vitamin D, 400 milligrams of magnesium and 300 milligrams of pantothenic acid (vitamin B5). Also, take 2 grams of distilled fish oil for omega-3 fatty acids and ½ teaspoon of cinnamon daily. And make sure you get 10 tablespoons of cooked tomato sauce weekly.
The Team	Don't be afraid to enlist advice from qualified nutritionists and trainers. But one of your most important team members will be your support partner – someone who can encourage you and be a deterrent to failure, too (you won't want to report to that person a four-doughnut binge).
The YOU-Turn	It's okay to make mistakes. The important thing is to catch them, recognize them, control them and allow yourself the opportunity to get back on the right (waist-management) road.

Eat to Stay Full – Not to Count Calories

Before we outline the meals, recipes and strategies for succeeding on the YOU Diet, we want you to remember this one principle of eating: eating isn't all about calories, it's about staying satisfied. The key to this programme is eating nutritionally rich foods, avoiding the toxic ones and using your body's clues about satiety to help you stop eating when you should.

It's about eating the foods that will help keep you full – and what 'feels right' – so that you can achieve and maintain your ideal playing weight. That said, we know some of you are members of the maths/stats/calorie squad, so we'll indulge your number-loving selves for a moment.

We've designed this diet and its serving sizes based on a person with a metabolic rate of 1,700 calories. That is, the person who burns 1,700 calories a day through normal processes and activities can eat this to maintain his or her weight. To lose weight, this person would have to have a slightly smaller portion for dinner, for instance. If you burn 2,000 calories a day, you'll lose weight using these portion sizes, but if you burn only 1,400 calories a day, you'll consume more calories than you burn. To find your approximate no-waist-loss point, find your resting metabolic rate and add your physical activities.

■ An easy way to estimate your resting metabolic rate is to multiply your desired weight in pounds by 8 and add 200, but this is very variable, so if anyone ever offers to measure your real metabolic rate, accept the offer.

■ To find the calories you burn from physical activity, multiply the number of minutes you walk by four, and your cardiovascular and strength minutes by eight. So that's about 300 calories for 30 minutes of walking and 25 minutes of strength or cardiovascular exercise. You can also use the readouts from cardiovascular machines you use if the machines have them.

So let's see how it works.

Say you want to weigh 150 pounds and do an average of 300 physical activity calories per day – about what you do on our plan (more on some days and fewer on others). That means:

Your basic calories used are 8 x 150 = 1,200
+ 200 = 1,400
+ 300 in activity = 1,700

So to maintain your desired weight, you'd need about 1,700 calories a day. To lose a pound a week, you'd need to decrease that by about 500 calories a day, or increase your physical activity by 500 calories a day, or a combination of the two. But tracking calories is a lot of work if you do not automate your eating. (There are also programs for handheld devices that can do it for you, such as at www.mychoicescount.com.) The point, though, isn't to track calories; it's to let your body, your stomach and your brain give you the signals to stop when you're satisfied, and not stuffed.

Be Prepared

Here's a waist-management fact: bad foods aren't bad just because of the ingredients they contain but also because many of them are fast and easy, which are the exact traits that can get you into a whole lot of trouble. The key to successful dietary contingency plans is to have premade foods ready for those times when you've been conditioned to reach for bags of sugar-containing waist killers. Instead, choose your favourites of these options to make once a week so you'll have something to grab when you need it.

Cut-up Vegetables: Your choice. Cut them, bag them, eat them. Try baby carrots, cherry tomatoes, broccoli florets, orange pepper strips ...

Sautéed Vegetables: Your choice. Sauté them in olive oil with chopped garlic, red pepper flakes or a good dash of turmeric. Refrigerate and use for side dishes or hot (microwaved) snacks.

The YOU Diet Meals: YOUR Choices

Below, we've listed your options for every food moment of the day (except dinner, which you'll find outlined specifically in the daily schedule). You can choose any of the options listed, but ideally choose just one or two to eat on most days. We've found that the most successful people are those who pick just one – and stick with it.

Soups: Make one or more of our filling YOU Soups (see recipes) once a week and store them in serving-size cups in the refrigerator. Eat one cup as a pre-dinner appetizer, to take the edge off, or have a cup of soup as a snack.

Steel-cut Oats: If you're worried about time, cook up one week's worth of oats per directions and store in the refrigerator for up to a week. For some people, that may seem as appetizing as a slice of baked wrapping paper, but reheated oats actually taste great.

Emergency Foods: Every house needs fire-extinguisher foods – good-for-you foods that will put out three-alarm starvation fires. Our list of foods that you can reach for when you're hungry include any of the above foods as well as a handful of almonds, peanuts or walnuts; bags of shop-bought, pre-chopped fruits and veggies; dried fruit (apricots, cranberries); and edamame (soya beans – look for microwave bags in the frozen food section). In a real pinch? Pop one of those mint breath strips – they can help turn off appetite by making food less appetizing.

YOUR Breakfast Choices

For Cereal Lovers

Cooked oat cereal with 115 ml of skimmed milk, or soya milk fortified with vitamin D and calcium, and 1 fistful of your favourite fruit, or

85 g Kashi high-fibre or cold-oat cereal (like Cheerios) with 1 fistful of your favourite fruit, with 115 ml of skimmed milk, or soya milk fortified with vitamin D and calcium

For Egg Lovers

Egg-white omelette (3 egg whites and 1 whole egg), plus cut-up mixed veggies, or

2 scrambled, poached or hard-boiled eggs with 2 pieces of lean turkey sausage or tofu sausage

For Bread Lovers

1 slice toasted wholewheat bread with 1 teaspoon peanut butter, or 1 teaspoon apple or walnut butter or avocado spread

For Breakfast Haters

Magical Breakfast Blaster (see recipe, page 277), or

Pineapple-banana Protein Blaster (see recipe, page 276)

YOUR Lunch Choices

Meal-size Salad

Chopped salad: 6 chopped walnuts, chopped veggies (your choice) and chopped mixed greens tossed with 115g of salmon, turkey or chicken breast; with balsamic vinegar (2 parts) and olive oil (1 part) dressing, or

One of the YOU Salads (recipes follow)

Soup and Salad

225g of one of the many hearty YOU Soups plus any of the YOU Salads (recipes for both follow) or a non-Caesar salad using olive or canola oil, or balsamic vinegar and olive oil dressing

Healthy Burger

Veggie burger or spicy chicken burger on a toasted wholewheat English muffin with 1 tablespoon of fructose-free olive oil-based marinara sauce, sliced tomato, romaine lettuce or spinach leaves, plus slices of red onion

YOUR Morning and Afternoon Snack Choices

Fruit and Nuts

15g raw nuts with an apple, banana, plum, pear, orange, wedge of melon, cup of berries, 2 kiwis, 1/2 grapefruit or any other fruit

Grains and Berries

30g whole-grain cereal mixed with 30g almonds and 30g dried berries, apricots or raisins

Revved-up Veggies

140g cut-up sautéed veggies, warmed in microwave and stuffed into small wholewheat pitta, or

Cut-up veggies dipped into 115g plain yogurt or low-fat cottage cheese mixed with lots of dill, chives, ginger, red pepper flakes or other spices (your choice), or

Just plain cut-up veggies

Fruit and Yogurt

Low-fat probiotic (live culture) yogurt covered with 115g of canned, unsweetened peaches or mandarin oranges and some raisins

YOUR Dessert Choices

Eat Every Other Day

Cinnamon-baked Apples with Tangerine and Cranberries (see recipe), or

Cinnamon Apple Sauté à la Mode (see recipe), or

Roasted Pear with Raspberry Coulis, Chocolate and Pistachios (see recipe), or

Sliced Peaches with Raspberries, Blueberries and Chocolate Chips (see recipe), or

1 ounce of dark chocolate (made with real cocoa),
approximately three or four bites

YOUR Evening Snack Choices
(But Don't Eat after 8.30pm)

Simon's Popcorn (see recipe), or

Any snack option, or

Wholewheat pitta toasts and Tomato-avocado Salsamole
(see recipe)

YOUR Drink Choices

Plain or sparkling water (with fruit slice if desired),
skimmed milk, coffee, hot or iced tea (decaffeinated is
best if you have problems sleeping), diet soda (but only 1
to 2 a day)

For breakfast, you may include a 225ml glass of fruit or
vegetable juice, such as tomato juice or 100 per cent
grapefruit juice or orange juice with pulp, fortified with
calcium and vitamin D

For dinner, you can include one glass of alcohol, which we prefer you to drink towards the end of the meal so it does not hinder your satiety centre's ability to slow your voracious appetite. If you're a non-drinker, it's okay to swap for a teetotaller's cocktail made with low-sugar grape juice, sparkling water and lime

The 14-day YOU Diet

By the end of the 14 days, you'll have developed eating patterns and behavioural habits that will help get you on your way to changing your body from the inside out. Here we outline the seven-day plan and strategies for making smart decisions about food and eating. In week two, you'll repeat the first week, making appropriate food substitutions where you wish.

Day One: Saturday

1. **Walk:** 30 minutes. Walking – whether you do it by yourself, with a friend, with your dog or around the dining room table – gives you your first dose of physical success. Walk every day for 30 minutes, and you'll establish the behavioural and motivational foundation for the YOU Diet.

2. **Stretch:** Do three to five minutes of stretching after your walk. See Chapter 11. Stretching not only keeps

your muscles flexible to help prevent injury, it also has a meditative element to it, helping you refocus and cope with cravings, as we explain on pages 215–16. 'No pain, no gain' does not apply here.

3. **Clear Out Your Fridge:** To make room for all the new, good food you're about to buy, it's time to rid your kitchen of the nutritional felons. The appeals are up; it's execution time. Read the label of everything in your kitchen cupboards, your refrigerator, your secret boxes and everywhere else you stash food. If something has any of the following in one of the first five ingredients, throw it out:

- Simple sugar. This includes brown sugar, dextrose, corn sweetener, fructose (as in high-fructose corn syrup), glucose, corn syrup, honey, invert sugar, maltose, lactose, malt syrup, molasses, raw sugar and sucrose. Keep a little table sugar handy, and honey and maple sugar, because you'll use some for recipes.
- Saturated fat. This includes most four-legged animal fat, milk fat, butter or lard and tropical oils, such as palm and coconut.
- Trans fat. This includes partially hydrogenated fats, vegetable oil blends that are hydrogenated and many margarines and cooking blends. (If you must, use cholesterol-fighting sterol spreads such as Benecol.)
- Enriched flours and all flours other than 100 per cent wholegrain or 100 per cent wholewheat. This includes enriched white flour, semolina, durum wheat and any of the acronyms for flour that is not wholewheat.

4. **Go Food Shopping:** The first week, you'll have a larger-than-normal shopping list because you'll stock up on essentials as well as ingredients you'll need for this week's recipes. For a specific shopping list that works with our suggested seven-day schedule, see page 267.

5. **Make Your Weekly Staples:** Your choice of vegetables or soup. See above.

Eat!

Follow guidelines for breakfast, lunch and snacks. For dinner, have …

Asian Salmon with Brown Rice Pilaf

Day Two: Sunday

1. **Walk:** 30 minutes.
2. **Stretch:** Do five minutes of stretching.
3. **Partner Up:** If you try to undertake this alone, there's a much higher risk that you'll end up lips-first in a tub of ice cream. Find your YOU partner – be it a spouse, a friend, a colleague – someone you can talk to about your goals, your meals, your new plan. Make a plan to talk (or email) five minutes every day – to tell them that you walked that day and about your day's meals. If you prefer a cyber friend, log on to www.realage.co.uk and match up with a partner there.

   Better yet, try to find a partner or partners who are in this *with* you. Share this book; share the knowledge you've learned; embark on a 'work smart, not hard' journey together.

Eat!

Follow guidelines for breakfast, lunch and snacks. For dinner, have ...

Spicy Chili or Stuffed Wholewheat Pizza

Day Three: Monday

1. **Walk:** 30 minutes. Start tightening your abs when you walk, which will help improve your posture and make your clothes fit better. Walk at a pace that raises your heart rate, or include 20 minutes of another cardiovascular exercise.

2. **Do the YOU Workout:** Follow the 20-minute no-weights YOU Workout, which includes both strength and stretching exercises, on page 220.

3. **Write it Down (or Type it in):** There's a fine line between guilt and motivation. One of the ways you can help reprogram yourself is by writing down everything that you eat. In a way, it holds you accountable; you won't want to eat bad foods, because you won't want the visual reminder that you ate them. For these two weeks only – just to establish your new routine – write down *everything* you eat. Yep, even the three M&Ms you just swiped. (For the technically savvy, some handheld devices have programs that allow you to scan the barcodes of the foods you eat. You enter the quantity

you eat, and the program will keep track of your calories
– see www.realage.co.uk or www.mychoicescount.com.)

4. **Go Shopping:** With three days of walking under your
soon-to-be-loose belt, it's time you made another trip
to the shops. This time, make it the sports shop – for a
good pair of running shoes. Use them for walking only.
If you like, you can also buy socks with extra padding
on the bottom (avoid cotton); a yoga mat, so you don't
slip and slide while enjoying the deep poses; dumbbells
or resistance bands if you're already advanced enough
to use those (see page 239).

Eat!

Follow guidelines for breakfast, lunch and snacks. For
dinner, have …

**Mediterranean Chicken with Tomato, Olives and
Herbed White Beans**

Day Four: Tuesday

1. **Walk:** 30 minutes.
2. **Stretch:** Do five minutes of stretching.
3. **Make Any Needed YOU-Turn:** It's not uncommon at
this point for you to have already dabbled in the neigh-
bour's cake or picked at the kids' chips. And that's okay.
Just get yourself back together.

At the next available moment, make an authorized
YOU-Turn.

Try these coping strategies:

- *The Lip Lick.* Breathe in, lick your lips, swallow and breathe out slowly, saying 'ohm'. Let the cool air flow across your lips. The soothing move – which takes all of about three seconds – helps you to reset, calm down and refocus.
- *The Waist Hang.* Stand up straight, bend over at your waist and let your lower back relax. Reach for the floor, grab your elbows or hold the back of your knees. The important thing is to let all of the tension you have stored in your back and hips unwind. Relax your neck completely. If you feel tight, don't straighten your knees.

Eat!

Follow guidelines for breakfast, lunch and snacks. For dinner, have ...

Royal Pasta Primavera Provençale

Day Five: Wednesday

1. **Walk:** 30 minutes.
2. **Do the YOU Workout:** Follow the 20-minute no-weights YOU Workout, which includes both strength and stretching exercises, on page 220.
3. **Call Your Doctor:** Remember, waist management is a team game, so schedule an appointment for 30 days from now (or sooner if you have a great relationship). You can use your doctor to help you in many different ways:

- Update your vitals such as blood pressure, waist size and heart rate. If you need a baseline for such numbers as HDL and LDL cholesterol (HDL is more important for women), now's a good time to book a medical, get a few blood tests and talk to your doctor about your new plan.
- Having a medical will also prove helpful when you reach a plateau – when your waist and weight loss seem to have stalled. (Your doctor may then be able to prescribe medication that can help you get over a hump.)

Eat!

Follow guidelines for breakfast, lunch and snacks. For dinner, have ...

Apricot Chicken and Green Beans with Almond Slivers

Day Six: Thursday

1. **Walk:** 30 minutes.
2. **Stretch:** Do five minutes of stretching.
3. **Do a Little Bragging:** If you go public with your success, it makes turning back more difficult. Tell a friend or a colleague about the progress you've made and the changes you've noticed.

Eat!

Follow guidelines for breakfast, lunch and snacks. For dinner, have ...

Turkey Tortilla Wraps with Red Baked Potato

Day Seven: Friday

1. **Walk:** 30 minutes.
2. **Do the YOU Workout:** Follow the 20-minute no-weights YOU Workout, which includes both strength and stretching exercises, on page 220.
3. **Restock Your Kitchen:** Check your cupboards for ingredients you've run out of and make a shopping list for next week's recipes.
4. **Grade Yourself:** Whether it's with work or a first date, it's always nice to have some way of knowing how you're progressing. Now is the time to take your waist measurement and weigh yourself, just to see what changes you've made. In your first week, you may see up to a one-inch waist reduction and a two- to four-pound weight reduction. You might even be able to drop one clothing size.

Eat!

Follow guidelines for breakfast, lunch and snacks. For dinner, have ...
Grilled Trout with Rosemary and Lemon

Day Eight to Forever: Your Reprogrammed Body

There you have it. We've given you all the tools, actions and adjustments you need to take your body back to its factory settings, with a healthy waist and a healthy weight. Now just repeat the steps for the second week, making meal substitutions as you like (see additional recipes starting on page 276). Work smart, not hard. Week one puts you in motion and allows your body to adjust. Week two gives you seven days to practise the plan, feel what it's like to eat well and work out what to do if you don't. Research shows that it takes two weeks of repetitive action to make the action become automated, so now you can take the plan and tweak it. Or repeat it. Or try new dinner recipes that you can find on our website, www.realage.co.uk. Make adjustments based on our nutritional guidelines as well as your tastes. This isn't the end of your waist-management plan; it's just the beginning.

When you reach a plateau – which you will – you have three choices: drop another few calories from your daily intake, increase your physical activity or see a doctor about extra help if appropriate. But remember that the purpose of losing weight is to gain health, so when you reach your playing weight and your body is loving the feeling, just stay the course.

Sample Eating Schedule

Want a plan that requires absolutely no thought at all? Then follow this schedule and the shopping list on page 267. *Note:* Because we all have higher or lower caloric needs, we do not dictate serving sizes here. Your goal is to eat the amount that makes you satisfied – that's a level three or four on our satiety scale (see pages 192–3), not feeling more bloated than a puffer fish.

Saturday

Breakfast: Cheerios with skimmed milk; juice and coffee or tea

Morning Snack: Yogurt with fruit

Lunch: Cup of Garden Harvest Soup; Cranberries, Walnuts and Crumbled Cheese over Greens

Afternoon Snack: Revved-up Veggies with dip

Dinner: Grilled Trout with Rosemary and Lemon; Rock Asparagus

Dessert: Cinnamon Apple Sauté à la Mode

Drinks: Water, coffee, tea, etc., as you wish

Sunday

Breakfast: Egg-white omelette; juice and coffee or tea

Morning Snack: Revved-up Veggies with dip

Lunch: Healthy Burger with the works

Afternoon Snack: Yogurt with fruit

Dinner: Asian Salmon with Brown Rice Pilaf

Dessert: 30g dark chocolate with orange slices

Drinks: Water, coffee, tea, etc., as you wish

Monday

Breakfast: Magical Breakfast Blaster
Morning Snack: 15g raw nuts
Lunch: Chopped salad of walnuts, veggies, greens and
   salmon/turkey/chicken
Afternoon Snack: Yogurt with fruit
Dinner: Stuffed Wholewheat Pizza
Evening Snack: Simon's Popcorn
Drinks: Water, coffee, tea, etc., as you wish

Tuesday

Breakfast: Cheerios with skimmed milk; juice and coffee
   or tea
Morning Snack: Apple
Lunch: Cup of Garden Harvest Soup; Cranberries, Walnuts
   and Crumbled Cheese over Greens
Afternoon Snack: Yogurt with fruit
Dinner: Mediterranean Chicken with Tomato, Olives and
   Herbed White Beans
Dessert: Cinnamon Apple Sauté à la Mode
Drinks: Water, coffee, tea, etc., as you wish

Wednesday

Breakfast: Magical Breakfast Blaster
Morning Snack: 30g raw nuts
Lunch: Chopped salad of walnuts, veggies, greens and
   salmon/turkey/chicken
Afternoon Snack: Yogurt and fruit
Dinner: Royal Pasta Primavera Provençale
Evening Snack: Tomato-avocado Salsamole and pitta
   toasts
Drinks: Water, coffee, tea, etc., as you wish

Thursday

Breakfast: Cheerios with skimmed milk; juice and coffee
   or tea
Morning Snack: Plum
Lunch: Cup of Garden Harvest Soup; Cranberries, Walnuts
   and Crumbled Cheese over Greens
Afternoon Snack: Revved-up Veggies in 1/2 wholewheat
   pitta
Dinner: Apricot Chicken and Green Beans with Almond
   Slivers
Dessert: 30g dark chocolate with a sliced orange
Drinks: Water, coffee, tea, etc., as you wish

Friday

Breakfast: Magical Breakfast Blaster
Morning Snack: 30g raw nuts
Lunch: Chopped salad of walnuts, veggies, greens and
    salmon/turkey/chicken
Afternoon Snack: Yogurt with fruit
Dinner: Turkey Tortilla Wraps with Red Baked Potato
Evening Snack: Simon's Popcorn
Drinks: Water, coffee, tea, etc., as you wish

Your Shopping List

The first week's shop will be the main one as you gather
the new building blocks for your fridge and cupboards
(including spices, oils and other long-term ingredients).
This list includes both your staples and your ingredients
for the recipes in our seven-day sample schedule, above.
You can make weekly or biweekly shopping lists for any of
the recipes and snack choices and for any number of
people (one to twenty-four) at www.realage.co.uk.

Shopping List Basics

Serves two for one week:

- The shopping list has been subdivided into categories to make shopping easier (grains, refrigerated items, protein, dried fruits and nuts, fresh veggies and so forth).
- A general condiment list has been included below for seasonings, spices, oils and so on, needed to complete the recipes. You may already have many of these items in your cupboards.
- Tomato or cranberry juice can be substituted for any or all of the orange juice.

Grains

1 box cold oat cereal (Cheerios)

1 packet 100 per cent wholewheat or 100 per cent wholegrain muffins or crumpets (try to find without sugar, honey or high-fructose corn syrup added)

One 12-inch or 10-ounce prepared thin 100 per cent whole-grain pizza crust

1 box short-grain brown rice

1 box 100 per cent wholewheat rigatoni or linguine pasta

1 box porridge oats

1 bag small 100 per cent wholewheat pittas

1 bag 100 per cent wholewheat tortillas

FACTOID

To ensure that a wholegrain food has a slower absorption in your digestive system and thus lowers your sugar and insulin levels, eat a little fat with it – in the form of ½ tablespoon of olive oil with your bread. Alternatively, eat six walnuts, 12 almonds or 20 peanuts about 20 minutes before you eat the wholegrain.

Canned/Jarred Items

1.8 litre low-salt vegetable or chicken stock or broth

1 tin (425–455g) white beans

2 tins (410g each) stewed tomatoes

1 tin whole, crushed or diced tomatoes

455g tomato sauce (with olive or canola oil and a low sugar content)

1 jar kalamata olives, halved

1 jar olive relish or tapenade

1 tin sun-dried tomato bits or finely chopped sun-dried tomatoes (not in oil)

2 tins unsweetened peaches or tangerines

1 small tin jalapeño peppers

1 jar popping corn

1 jar unsweetened apple juice or cider (preferably organic)

1 jar apple butter (keep in fridge)

1 jar all-natural peanut butter (no trans fat, no added sugar or fructose)

Dried Fruits and Nuts

1 bag raw walnuts (at least 225g)
1 bag raw hazelnuts (at least 115g)
1 bag raw almonds (at least 115g)
1 bag slivered almonds
1 bag dried cranberries
1 bag dried apricots
1 packet chopped pistachios (enough for 1 1/2
    tablespoons)

Staple Condiments/Spices

Buy these or make sure you have them in your cupboards.
Refill as needed.

Olive oil
Canola oil
Salt
Pepper
Fresh garlic
Low-sodium soy sauce
Balsamic vinegar
Wine vinegar
Maple syrup (look for a brand that doesn't have high-
    fructose corn syrup listed in the first four
    ingredients)
Marinara sauce or other red tomato sauce
Dijon mustard
Hot red pepper sauce

Nutmeg

Cinnamon

Your favourite coffee or tea

Dark chocolate bar with at least 70 per cent cocoa, or 1
small bag mini semi-sweet all-cocoa chocolate chips
(not milk chocolate and without milk fat)

Refrigerated Items

4 pints skimmed milk or low-fat soya milk fortified with
calcium and vitamin D

2 pints 100 per cent orange or grapefruit juice with pulp,
fortified with calcium, magnesium and vitamin D

170g crumbled farmer cheese

6 eggs

1 bag finely shredded low-fat mozzarella cheese (enough
for 55g)

8 x 115g containers of probiotic low-fat yogurt

Chicken/Turkey/Fish

2 bone-in chicken thighs without skin

2 skinless, boneless chicken breast halves (about 115g each)

340g sliced cooked salmon (or white turkey or chicken
from deli)

225g skinless salmon fillets (or skinless chicken or turkey
breasts)

1 whole fish (such as trout, about 115g per serving)

Frozen Food

1 box spicy chicken burgers
1 bag frozen unsweetened blueberries
1 bag frozen unsweetened raspberries
1 small container fat-free or low-fat vanilla frozen yogurt

Health Food Aisle or Health Food Store

Soya protein
Psyllium
Flaxseed

Other

1 bottle white wine

Fruit and Veg (shop last)

Wild Card: If you especially like particular fruits or
   vegetables, buy them in whatever quantities you want
   and eat them as substitutions or additions to your
   recipes (especially in season).
3 x 285g bags of salad mix (classic romaine or other
   mixed-green salad)
795g mixed mesclun or spring greens
455g cut-up stir-fry veggies (asparagus, broccoli,
   cauliflower, mushrooms, multicoloured peppers, red
   and white onions, courgettes)
Sliced carrots, apples, broccoli and/or celery in a packet

900g other veggies (your choice) to sauté, dip, mix into
    omelettes, chop into salads
5 small apples
2 small plums
3 tomatoes
1 bunch of carrots
1 bunch of bananas
2 red peppers
1 yellow or orange pepper
1 small head cabbage
85g beans
455g asparagus spears
1 small aubergine
3 shallots
2 large cloves garlic
3 medium yellow onions
1 red onion
1 small bunch of green onions
1 small dried ancho or pasilla chili pepper
1 large russet baking potato
1 bunch each fresh parsley, basil, rosemary, thyme (or
    lemon thyme), chives, oregano and chervil
1 piece root ginger
1 lime
1 avocado
1 small punnet fresh raspberries (if available; if not,
    substitute frozen)
1 small punnet fresh blueberries (if available; if not,
    substitute frozen)

Restaurant Tricks

Eating out can be a great experience — for everyone except your gut.
While you should always follow our guidelines for good foods (the waist
foods, not the waste foods, in our crib sheet), you should also know that
most dietary mistakes are made within the first and last 10 minutes of
any restaurant experience. Some tips:

- Return the free bread and ask if you can have cut-up raw vegetables
  instead. (Do this four times in a three-week period, and we've found
  that most good restaurants remember the trick and automatically
  make that change every time they see you — if they see you at least
  once a week.)
- Order oil and vinegar in separate containers and on the side for salad
  dressing, and put a little on. (You have to do this; relying on the
  waiter or chef to do so gets you about 400 extra calories per side
  salad.)
- Ask to replace the potato or rice with sautéed vegetables.
- If you're going to have dessert, order one for the table and have just
  a few bites.

The YOU Diet Troubleshooting Guide

If YOU ...	Then YOU ...
Eat something you shouldn't	Don't worry, but don't keep eating. Use one of our YOU-Turn techniques (a stretch, a meditation technique or the lip lick) to refocus so you don't turn one mistake into a buffet-clearing gorge.
Stall with weight/waist loss	Talk to your doctor about using medication to help you get past the plateau to lead to further weight/waist loss.
Can't find a support partner	If you can't blackmail a partner with all the benefits she'll also receive (she too will learn about elegant solutions she can apply to her own life), then match yourself with one at www.realage.co.uk.
Have a family that decides to go out for a buffet meal tonight	Before you go, have a cup of soup, a handful of nuts and one glass of water. That will fill you up before you eat, so you eat sensibly and automatically. And limit yourself to one trip with a seven- or nine-inch plate, and keep it to single-storey servings.
Feel foot pain and find it hard to walk	Stop walking and find an alternative activity such as biking or swimming. See a podiatrist to diagnose your ailment.

Travel all the time and have to eat on the road a lot	Rely on more snacks rather than gorging on big meals. Travel with easy-to-carry (in plastic bags) snacks such as nuts and cut-up apples and carrots to take the edge off your hunger.
Are diagnosed with a serious illness	It's not always the time to lose weight when you're sick, but it is the ideal time to get food on your side. But if you're prescribed a drug that may slow weight loss (like a beta-blocker), talk to your doctor about a more aggressive weight-loss approach that's ailment-appropriate, since subsequent weight loss is more difficult.
Might have a food allergy (for example, irritable bowel syndrome or unexplained lethargy)	Do the elimination diet found on page 96.

The YOU Diet Recipes

YOU Drinks

Pineapple-Banana Protein Blaster

2 servings • 207 calories per serving

1 large ripe banana
115ml low-fat soya milk
115g tinned crushed pineapple in juice, undrained
115g 'pineapple-passion' sorbet, such as Select brand (a
    Safeway brand)
1 tablespoon soya protein powder (8 grams protein)

Peel banana; break into chunks. Combine all ingredients in blender. Cover; blend until fairly smooth.

What's in it for you?

Total fat	2g	Carbohydrates	38g	Calcium	39mg
Saturated fat	0.8g	Sugar	17g	Magnesium	40mg
Healthy fats	1.1g	Protein	11g	Selenium	1mcg
Fibre	2.1g	Sodium	31mg	Potassium	428mg

Magical Breakfast Blaster

2 servings • 136 calories per serving

½ large ripe banana (or other fruit of your choice)
1 scoop (85g) soya protein (like Nature's Plus Spiru-Tein:
    naturesplus.com)
½ tablespoon flaxseed oil
45g frozen blueberries
½ tablespoon apple juice concentrate or honey
1 teaspoon psyllium seed husks
225ml water

Peel banana; break into chunks. Combine all ingredients in a blender. Optional: add a few cubes of ice, as well as powdered vitamins. Cover; blend until fairly smooth.

What's in it for you?

Total fat	2.6g	Carbohydrates	16.8g	Calcium	93.5mg
Saturated fat	0.3g	Sugar	11.1g	Magnesium	33.1mg
Healthy fats	2.4g	Protein	29g	Selenium	1.8mcg
Fibre	6.3g	Sodium	380mg	Potassium	195mg

YOU Soups

Garden Harvest Soup

10 servings • 176 calories per serving

1 tablespoon olive oil

1 medium onion, chopped

1 carrot, chopped

4 garlic cloves, thinly sliced

1 red pepper, chopped

1.8 litre low-salt vegetable or chicken stock or broth

795g tinned whole, crushed or diced tomatoes, undrained

450ml water

1 small head cabbage, thinly sliced

½ teaspoon hot red pepper sauce (optional)

Salt and freshly ground black pepper (optional)

Optional garnishes: chopped fresh parsley, chopped fresh
    coriander

Heat a large saucepan over medium-high heat. Add oil, then onion; cook 5 minutes, stirring occasionally. Stir in carrot, garlic and pepper; cook until tender. Add stock, tomatoes, water and cabbage; simmer uncovered 20 minutes. Season to taste with hot sauce and salt and pepper if desired. Garnish with parsley or coriander if desired.

What's in it for you?

Total fat	4g	Carbohydrates	15.9g	Calcium	73mg
Saturated fat	0.8g	Sugar	4.6g	Magnesium	35mg
Healthy fats	2.85g	Protein	7.1g	Selenium	5.6mcg
Fibre	3.6g	Sodium	374mg	Potassium	631mg

Lisa's Great Gazpacho

4 servings • 120 calories per serving

795g tinned crushed or diced tomatoes, undrained

225ml tomato juice

115g each: diced (¼ inch) red or orange pepper, unpeeled
   cucumber

30g red onion, finely chopped

2 green onions, finely chopped

1 bunch coriander leaves, chopped

3 tablespoons red wine vinegar or apple cider vinegar

3 tablespoons extra-virgin olive oil

2 dashes (or to taste) hot red pepper sauce

2 garlic cloves, grated

Salt and freshly ground black pepper (optional)

Optional garnishes: chopped fresh parsley, diced avocado

Place all ingredients except salt, pepper and garnishes in large bowl and combine. Coarsely purée about half the mixture in a blender or food processor and return it to the bowl; stir well. Season to taste with salt and pepper if desired. Refrigerate for at least 2 hours and up to 8 hours before serving. Garnish as desired.

What's in it for you?

Total fat	12.1g	Carbohydrates	19.2g	Calcium	74mg
Saturated fat	1.8g	Sugar	5.2g	Magnesium	53mg
Healthy fats	10.2g	Protein	4.4g	Selenium	0.9mcg
Fibre	4.6g	Sodium	207mg	Potassium	780mg

Spicy Vegetable Lentil Soup

10 servings • 94 calories per serving

1 tablespoon olive oil

1 medium onion, chopped

1 carrot, chopped

1 red pepper, chopped

5 garlic cloves, sliced

1.8 litres water

200g dried lentils

795g tinned crushed tomatoes, undrained

2 bay leaves

2 tablespoons balsamic vinegar

Salt and freshly ground black pepper (optional)

Heat oil in a large saucepan over medium-high heat. Add onion; cook 5 minutes, stirring occasionally. Stir in carrot, pepper and garlic; cook 3 minutes. Stir in remaining ingredients except salt and pepper; bring to a boil over high heat. Reduce heat; simmer uncovered 18 to 20 minutes, or until lentils and vegetables are tender. Season to taste with salt and pepper if desired. Remove bay leaves before serving.

What's in it for you?

Total fat	1.6g	Carbohydrates	8g	Calcium	26mg
Saturated fat	0.2g	Sugar	1.6g	Magnesium	16mg
Healthy fats	1.4g	Protein	1.9g	Selenium	0.6mcg
Fibre	2.8g	Sodium	82mg	Potassium	228mg

Two-onion Delight

8 servings • 129 calories per serving

1 tablespoon olive oil
2 onions, sliced
2 shallots, sliced
1 leek (white and light-green part only), sliced
1.8 litres low-salt chicken stock or broth
Salt and freshly ground black pepper (optional)
115g grated low-fat Swiss cheese
1 bunch chives, finely chopped

Heat oil in a large saucepan over medium-high heat. Add onions; cook 5 minutes, stirring occasionally. Stir in shallots and leek; continue cooking until golden brown, about 5 minutes. Add stock; simmer uncovered 15 minutes. Season to taste with salt and pepper if desired. Ladle into shallow bowls; garnish with cheese and chives.

What's in it for you?

Total fat	5g	Carbohydrates	12.3g	Calcium	84mg
Saturated fat	1.2g	Sugar	5.7g	Magnesium	16mg
Healthy fats	3.4g	Protein	8.5g	Selenium	6.4mcg
Fibre	0.3g	Sodium	385mg	Potassium	321mg

Curried Split Pea Soup

8 servings • 155 calories per serving

1 tablespoon olive oil
1 onion, chopped
1 carrot, chopped
4 garlic cloves, sliced
920ml low-salt vegetable stock or broth
920ml water
200g dried yellow split peas
1 teaspoon curry powder
1 teaspoon ground cumin
½ bunch parsley, chopped

Heat oil in a large saucepan over medium-high heat. Add onion; cook 5 minutes, stirring occasionally. Add carrot and garlic; cook until softened, about 5 minutes. Add remaining ingredients except parsley; bring to a boil. Reduce heat; simmer uncovered 30 minutes, or until peas are tender. Ladle into shallow bowls; garnish with parsley.

What's in it for you?

Total fat	3.6g	Carbohydrates	22g	Calcium	30.8mg
Saturated fat	0.7g	Sugar	5.1g	Magnesium	38mg
Healthy fats	2.7g	Protein	9.5g	Selenium	3.4mcg
Fibre	6.8g	Sodium	183mg	Potassium	432mg

Quick Black Bean Soup

8 servings • 445 calories per serving

1 tablespoon olive oil

1 onion, chopped

3 garlic cloves, sliced

1 carrot, chopped

2 stalks celery, chopped

1.8 litres low-salt vegetable stock or broth

850–900g tinned black beans, rinsed and drained

1 teaspoon ground coriander

¼ teaspoon cayenne pepper

1 tablespoon balsamic vinegar

1 bunch coriander leaves, chopped

Heat oil in a large saucepan over medium-high heat. Add onion; cook 5 minutes, stirring occasionally. Add garlic, carrot and celery; cook until soft, about 5 minutes. Add stock, beans, coriander and cayenne pepper; simmer uncovered 10 minutes. Stir in vinegar. Transfer to blender or food processor; process to desired consistency. Reheat if necessary. Ladle into shallow bowls; garnish with coriander.

What's in it for you?

Total fat	6g	Carbohydrates	71.8g	Calcium	139mg
Saturated fat	1.4g	Sugar	7.4g	Magnesium	180mg
Healthy fats	2.8g	Protein	27.4g	Selenium	1mcg
Fibre	15.3g	Sodium	360mg	Potassium	1,771mg

Minted Fresh Pea Soup

8 servings • 157 calories per serving

1 tablespoon olive oil

1 onion, chopped

1 carrot, chopped

2 garlic cloves, grated

285g frozen or fresh peas

1.8 litres low-salt vegetable stock or broth

225g low-fat plain yogurt

Salt and freshly ground black pepper (optional)

1 small bunch mint leaves, chopped

Heat oil in a large saucepan over medium-high heat. Add onion; cook 5 minutes, stirring occasionally. Add carrot and garlic; cook until soft, about 5 minutes. Add peas and stock; simmer uncovered 20 minutes. Transfer in batches to blender or food processor and add yogurt; purée until smooth. Season to taste with salt and pepper if desired. Reheat if needed; ladle into shallow bowls; garnish with mint.

What's in it for you?

Total fat	4.8g	Carbohydrates	18.2g	Calcium	84mg
Saturated fat	1.1g	Sugar	9.5g	Magnesium	30.3mg
Healthy fats	3.5g	Protein	10g	Selenium	7.3mcg
Fibre	2.3g	Sodium	376mg	Potassium	466mg

YOU Salads

Japanese Ginger Salad with Pumpkin Seeds and Sprouts

8 servings • 230 calories per serving

Dressing Ingredients

115ml olive oil

115ml rice vinegar

1 small sweet onion, quartered

1 large carrot, chopped

1 tablespoon orange juice

1 tablespoon grated fresh ginger

¼ teaspoon soy sauce

Salt and freshly ground black pepper (optional)

Salad Ingredients

2 large heads romaine lettuce, torn

45g fresh bean sprouts

30g pumpkin seeds

Combine all dressing ingredients except salt and pepper in blender or food processor; purée until smooth. Season to taste with salt and pepper if desired. Toss lettuce with dressing; top with sprouts and seeds.

What's in it for you?

Total fat	22g	Sugar	4g	Magnesium	74mg
Healthy fats	12.1g	Protein	6.4g	Selenium	2mcg
Fibre	6g	Sodium	53mg	Potassium	499mg
Carbohydrates	16.8g	Calcium	79mg		

Spinach-walnut-citrus Salad

2 servings • 246 calories per serving

Dressing Ingredients
1 tablespoon olive oil
1 tablespoon white wine vinegar
1 teaspoon honey
Dash of cayenne pepper
Salt and freshly ground black pepper (optional)

Salad Ingredients
1 large bunch spinach, washed and trimmed
20g walnut halves, raw or pan-roasted (beware of smoke-
    detector sounds if you do this like Dr Mike and answer the
    phone when it rings only to forget what is in pan roasting)
½ orange, cut into segments
½ grapefruit, cut into segments
2 green onions, chopped

Combine oil, vinegar, honey and cayenne pepper; mix well. Season to taste with salt and pepper if desired. Toss spinach with dressing and walnuts. Arrange orange and grapefruit sections on top and garnish with green onions.

What's in it for you?

Total fat	17g	Carbohydrates	21g	Calcium	218mg
Saturated fat	1.9g	Sugar	7.6g	Magnesium	169mg
Healthy fats	14.4g	Protein	8g	Selenium	3.6mcg
Fibre	6.8g	Sodium	138mg	Potassium	1,203mg

Cranberries, Walnuts and Crumbled Cheese over Greens

2 servings • 304 calories per serving

Dressing Ingredients

1 tablespoon olive oil

1 tablespoon balsamic vinegar

½ teaspoon Dijon mustard

1 garlic clove, grated

¼ teaspoon soy sauce

Salt and freshly ground black pepper (optional)

Salad Ingredients

285g packed mixed greens

30g dried cranberries

20g walnut halves, raw or pan-roasted

55g crumbled farmer cheese

Combine oil, vinegar, mustard, garlic and soy sauce; mix well. Season to taste with salt and pepper if desired. Toss greens with dressing, cranberries and walnuts. Arrange on serving plates; top with cheese.

What's in it for you?

Total fat	22.7g	Carbohydrates	19.6g	Calcium	146mg
Saturated fat	6g	Sugar	11.9g	Magnesium	57mg
Healthy fats	15.6g	Protein	10g	Selenium	3mcg
Fibre	4.7g	Sodium	183mg	Potassium	391mg

Rocket, Watermelon and Feta Salad

2 servings • 190 calories per serving

Dressing Ingredients
1 tablespoon olive oil
1 tablespoon balsamic vinegar
1 small shallot, grated
Salt and freshly ground black pepper (optional)

Salad Ingredients
1 large bunch of rocket, washed and dried
170g cubed seedless watermelon
55g crumbled low-fat feta cheese

Combine oil, vinegar and shallot; mix well. Season to taste with salt and pepper if desired; let stand 5 minutes. Arrange rocket on 2 serving plates. Arrange watermelon and cheese on top of rocket; drizzle with dressing.

What's in it for you?

Total fat	13.3g	Carbohydrates	13g	Calcium	235mg
Saturated fat	5.3g	Sugar	6.9g	Magnesium	41.8mg
Healthy fats	7.3g	Protein	6.4g	Selenium	5mcg
Fibre	1.1g	Sodium	334mg	Potassium	377mg

Turkish Shepherd Salad

2 servings • 153 calories per serving

1 small cucumber
1 tomato
1 small sweet onion
1 teaspoon olive oil
1 tablespoon red wine vinegar
Salt and freshly ground black pepper (optional)
55g crumbled low-fat feta cheese

Coarsely chop cucumber, tomato and onion; transfer to a bowl. Add oil and vinegar; toss well. Season to taste with salt and pepper if desired. Transfer to serving plates; top with cheese.

What's in it for you?

Total fat	8.6g	Carbohydrates	14.7g	Calcium	186mg
Saturated fat	4.6g	Sugar	9g	Magnesium	39mg
Healthy fats	3.6g	Protein	6.1g	Selenium	5.1mcg
Fibre	2.2g	Sodium	329mg	Potassium	479mg

Greek Feta Salad with Peppers and Olives

2 servings • 305 calories per serving

Dressing Ingredients

1 tablespoon olive oil

1 tablespoon red wine vinegar

1 tablespoon lemon juice

½ teaspoon dried oregano

1 garlic clove, grated

½ teaspoon honey

Salt and freshly ground black pepper (optional)

Salad Ingredients

1 head romaine lettuce, torn

1 tomato, quartered

4 pepperoncini peppers

1 small cucumber, sliced

55g crumbled low-fat feta cheese

Several sprigs fresh dill, chopped

½ green pepper, sliced into rings

8 kalamata olives

Combine all dressing ingredients except salt and pepper; mix well. Season to taste with salt and pepper if desired; let stand 5 minutes. Combine all salad ingredients in large bowl; toss with dressing.

What's in it for you?

Total fat	16g	Carbohydrates	35.8g	Calcium	324mg
Saturated fat	5.7g	Sugar	17.9g	Magnesium	108mg
Healthy fats	9.6g	Protein	12g	Selenium	619mcg
Fibre	10.9g	Sodium	510mg	Potassium	1,593mg

Orient Express Salad with Chopped Peanuts

2 servings • 200 calories per serving

Dressing Ingredients

1 tablespoon olive oil

2 tablespoons orange juice

1 tablespoon rice wine vinegar

1 teaspoon grated fresh root ginger

1 teaspoon soy sauce

½ teaspoon toasted sesame oil

Salt and freshly ground black pepper (optional)

Salad Ingredients

2 small heads lettuce, torn

1 small cucumber, sliced

1 small bunch coriander, coarsely chopped

1 carrot, shredded

2 tablespoons chopped peanuts

2 green onions, chopped

Combine all dressing ingredients except salt and pepper; mix well. Season to taste with salt and pepper if desired. Toss lettuce, cucumber, coriander and carrot with the dressing. Transfer to serving plates; top with peanuts and green onions.

What's in it for you?

Total fat	13.1g	Carbohydrates	17.7g	Calcium	121mg
Saturated fat	1.8g	Sugar	7.9g	Magnesium	72mg
Healthy fats	10.6g	Protein	7.1g	Selenium	2.3mcg
Fibre	5.1g	Sodium	458mg	Potassium	936mg

Sweet Beet and Gorgonzola Salad

4 servings • 106 calories per serving

6 medium beets, trimmed

1 tablespoon olive oil

1 tablespoon balsamic vinegar

1 teaspoon honey

1 garlic clove, pressed or grated

½ teaspoon soy sauce

½ bunch of chives, finely chopped

2 tablespoons crumbled Gorgonzola cheese

In large saucepan, simmer beets in water to cover until tender but still firm, about 30 minutes. Drain, cool and remove skin. Meanwhile, combine oil, vinegar, honey, garlic and soy sauce in a medium bowl. Cut beets into 1-inch cubes; add to bowl. Toss with dressing and chives. Transfer to serving plates; top with cheese.

What's in it for you?

Total fat	4.8g	Carbohydrates	13.7g	Calcium	45mg
Saturated fat	1.3g	Sugar	9.8g	Magnesium	31mg
Healthy fats	3.3g	Protein	3.1g	Selenium	1.6mcg
Fibre	3.5g	Sodium	239mg	Potassium	424mg

Mediterranean Cauliflower Salad

4 servings • 94 calories per serving

1 head cauliflower, blanched for 5 minutes

1 small tin anchovies, drained, chopped (optional)

1 tablespoon drained capers

2 tablespoons fresh lemon juice

1 tablespoon olive oil

1 garlic clove, pressed or grated

1 tablespoon chopped fresh oregano or 1 teaspoon dried

Drain cauliflower and break into small pieces. Combine cauliflower, anchovies if desired and capers in a medium bowl. Combine remaining ingredients; toss with cauliflower mixture.

What's in it for you?

Total fat	4.6g	Carbohydrates	8.8g	Calcium	63mg
Saturated fat	0.7g	Sugar	3.7g	Magnesium	31mg
Healthy fats	3.7g	Protein	6.2g	Selenium	8.7mcg
Fibre	3.8g	Sodium	519mg	Potassium	514mg

Hearts of Palm Salad with Tomato and Mushrooms

2 servings • 132 calories per serving

455g tinned hearts of palm, drained
1 tomato, chopped
1 shallot, chopped
6 button mushrooms, sliced
1 small bunch parsley, chopped
2 tablespoons red wine vinegar
1 tablespoon olive oil
Salt and freshly ground black pepper (optional)

Slice hearts of palm in half lengthwise; arrange on a serving platter. Combine remaining ingredients except salt and pepper; mix well. Season to taste with salt and pepper if desired. Spoon mixture over hearts of palm.

What's in it for you?

Total fat	8g	Carbohydrates	12.2g	Calcium	102mg
Saturated fat	1.2g	Sugar	2.6g	Magnesium	72mg
Healthy fats	6.2g	Protein	6.2g	Selenium	6mcg
Fibre	5g	Sodium	632mg	Potassium	632mg

Carrot, Raisin and Yogurt Slaw

2 servings • 193 calories per serving

4 carrots, shredded
1 small bunch coriander, chopped
225g low-fat Greek-style yogurt
30g raisins
1 garlic clove, grated
1 teaspoon lemon juice
Dash of Worcestershire sauce
Salt and freshly ground black pepper (optional)

Combine all ingredients except salt and pepper in a bowl; mix well. Season to taste with salt and pepper if desired.

What's in it for you?

Total fat	4.5g	Carbohydrates	35g	Calcium	2.5mg
Saturated fat	2.7g	Sugar	23g	Magnesium	41mg
Healthy fats	1.4g	Protein	6.5g	Selenium	3.3mcg
Fibre	5.1g	Sodium	166mg	Potassium	850mg

Sesame Cucumber Salad

2 servings • 187 calories per serving

1 tablespoon rice wine vinegar
1 teaspoon olive oil
½ teaspoon toasted sesame oil
½ teaspoon soy sauce
Dash cayenne pepper
2 cucumbers, cut into ¼-inch-thick slices
½ bunch chives, grated
1 teaspoon sesame seeds

Combine vinegar, olive oil, sesame oil, soy sauce and cayenne pepper in a medium bowl; mix well. Add cucumbers, chives and sesame seeds; mix well.

What's in it for you?

Total fat	6.8g	Carbohydrates	29g	Calcium	90mg
Saturated fat	1g	Sugar	8.2g	Magnesium	85mg
Healthy fats	5.3g	Protein	6.2g	Selenium	18.1mcg
Fibre	3.2g	Sodium	180mg	Potassium	750mg

YOU Dinners

Asian Salmon with Brown Rice Pilaf

4 servings • 674 calories per serving

Brown Rice

1 tablespoon olive oil

½ onion, chopped

½ red pepper, chopped

450ml water

200g uncooked short-grain brown rice

15g finely chopped parsley

Salt and freshly ground black pepper (optional)

Salmon Ingredients

4 skinless salmon fillets (about 115g each)

1 tablespoon olive oil

1 garlic clove, pressed or grated

1 tablespoon grated fresh root ginger

1 teaspoon soy sauce

1 teaspoon maple syrup

2 green onions, chopped

To make the rice, heat oil in a medium saucepan. Add onion and pepper; cook 3 minutes. Add water and rice; bring to a boil. Reduce heat; cover and simmer 50 minutes, or until rice is tender and liquid is absorbed. Fluff with a fork; stir in parsley. Season with salt and pepper if desired. Meanwhile, place salmon in a pie plate or shallow dish. Combine remaining salmon ingredients; mix well. Pour marinade over salmon; let stand 15 to 20 minutes. Heat a ridged grill pan over medium heat until hot. Add salmon, discarding marinade; cook 3 to 4 minutes per side, or until salmon is opaque and firm to the touch. Serve with brown rice.

What's in it for you?

Total fat	20.5g	Carbohydrates	45.9g	Calcium	81mg
Saturated fat	3.4g	Sugar	4.9g	Magnesium	165mg
Healthy fats	15g	Protein	71g	Selenium	145mcg
Fibre	2.6g	Sodium	411mg	Potassium	1,421mg

Spicy Chili

4 servings • 390 calories per serving

1 tablespoon olive oil
225g minced turkey or meat substitute (such as Quorn)
½ onion, chopped
2 garlic cloves, grated
795g tinned crushed tomatoes, undrained
455g tinned kidney beans, drained
½ teaspoon chili powder
Pinch of cayenne pepper
1 teaspoon maple syrup
1 teaspoon wine vinegar
½ teaspoon ground coriander
½ teaspoon turmeric
Brown Rice Pilaf (recipe on page 308)

Heat oil in a large saucepan. Add turkey, onion and garlic; cook 5 minutes, stirring frequently. Add remaining ingredients; simmer uncovered 25 minutes. Serve over Brown Rice Pilaf.

What's in it for you?

Total fat	8.9g	Carbohydrates	31.5g	Calcium	86mg
Saturated fat	1.9g	Sugar	2.2g	Magnesium	73mg
Healthy fats	6.2g	Protein	18.8g	Selenium	13.3mcg
Fibre	10.7g	Sodium	646mg	Potassium	838mg

Trust Crust

To bake your own wholewheat pizza crust, the recipe will require 25 to 70 extra minutes from start to finish, including time for yeast to do its thing. In a small bowl, combine about 1 tablespoon of dry yeast and ⅛ teaspoon of sugar with 340ml of warm water. Let that sit for 10 minutes. In a separate large bowl, combine 200g wholewheat flour and 200g plain (enriched) flour. (After you've tried this on your family several times, you can gradually increase in 65g lots the ratio of wholewheat to plain flour to 330g wholewheat to 70g plain.) Add 1 teaspoon sea salt to this. Mix well. Then add the yeast mixture and mix by hand thoroughly. Add 1 tablespoon olive oil. Knead for about 2 minutes until dough is smooth. Cover bowl and let rise in warm area until dough has doubled in size (20 to 60 minutes). Punch down dough with your fist and knead for 1 to 2 minutes. Divide into 4 equal portions (extra portions can be stored in your refrigerator). Roll into balls and preheat oven to 450°F/230°C/GM8. Lightly coat a baking sheet with olive oil. With a rolling pin, roll one of dough balls on rolling board or on baking sheet (add flour if dough sticks to pin too much) and flatten into 10–12-inch pizza crust circle. Poke with a fork 4 to 6 times. Bake for 5 minutes. Remove from oven, then add ingredients.

Stuffed Wholewheat Pizza

4 servings (2 slices per serving); for the first two weeks, you can have up to half of the pizza, but most will not need that much to be filled • 322 calories per serving

Cooking oil spray
455g fresh stir-fry vegetables such as asparagus, broccoli,
      cauliflower, mushrooms, multicoloured peppers, red and
      white onions and courgettes, cut up
2 garlic cloves, grated
Salt and freshly ground black pepper (optional)
225ml pizza sauce or tomato sauce
2 tablespoons olive relish or tapenade
2 tablespoons sun-dried-tomato bits
One 12-inch or 285g prepared thin wholewheat pizza crust
55g finely grated low-fat mozzarella cheese

Heat oven to 425°F/220°C/GM7. Heat a large nonstick frying pan over medium-high heat until hot; coat with cooking spray. Add vegetables and garlic; stir-fry (really sauté) 2 to 5 minutes, or until vegetables are crisp-tender. Season to taste with salt and pepper if desired. Combine pizza sauce, olive relish and sun-dried-tomato bits. Spread over pizza crust; top with cooked vegetables and cheese. Bake pizza directly on oven rack 10 to 15 minutes, or until crust is golden brown and cheese is melted. Cut pizza into 8 wedges.

What's in it for you?

Total fat	11.5g	Carbohydrates	44.2g	Calcium	151mg
Saturated fat	3.5g	Sugar	3.5g	Magnesium	44mg
Healthy fats	7.9g	Protein	12.2g	Selenium	2.9mcg
Fibre	5.7g	Sodium	682mg	Potassium	481mg

Mediterranean Chicken with Tomatoes, Olives and Herbed White Beans

2 servings • 567 calories per serving

Chicken Ingredients

2 bone-in chicken thighs without skin

1 tomato, chopped

½ onion, chopped

8 pitted kalamata olives, halved

1 tablespoon olive oil

1 teaspoon wine vinegar or balsamic vinegar

1 small bunch fresh basil, chopped

Bean Ingredients

1 tablespoon olive oil

2 garlic cloves, grated

425–455g tinned white beans, rinsed and drained

1 tomato, chopped

15g chopped fresh mixed herbs

1 teaspoon red wine vinegar or balsamic vinegar

Salt and freshly ground black pepper (optional)

To make the chicken, heat oven to 375°F/190°C/GM5. Place each chicken thigh on a large square of aluminium foil. Combine remaining chicken ingredients; spoon over chicken. Fold foil up and over chicken, sealing edges and forming a packet. Bake 25 minutes, or until chicken is cooked through. Meanwhile, to prepare the beans, heat oil in a medium saucepan over medium heat. Add garlic; cook 2 minutes. Add remaining bean ingredients; cook 5 minutes, or until heated through. Carefully open chicken packets and transfer mixture to two serving plates; serve beans alongside chicken.

What's in it for you?

Total fat	19.2g	Carbohydrates	67.4g	Calcium	243mg
Saturated fat	3.1g	Sugar	5.1g	Magnesium	171mg
Healthy fats	15g	Protein	34.4g	Selenium	14.3mcg
Fibre	15.2g	Sodium	313mg	Potassium	1,715mg

Royal Pasta Primavera Provençale

2 servings • 451 calories per serving

170g wholewheat rigatoni or linguine pasta

1 small dried chili pepper

115g diced (½-inch cubes) unpeeled aubergine

1 teaspoon olive oil

1 small yellow onion, coarsely chopped

1 yellow or orange pepper, coarsely chopped

3 garlic cloves, sliced

825g tinned stewed tomatoes, undrained, coarsely chopped

85g mixed salad greens

1 teaspoon chopped fresh thyme or lemon thyme

Salt and freshly ground black pepper (optional)

Cook pasta according to packet directions, omitting salt and fat. Meanwhile, heat a large, deep frying pan over medium heat until hot. Add the chili pepper; cook, turning occasionally until fragrant and toasted, about 2 minutes. When the chili pepper is cool enough to handle, discard its stem and set the seeds aside for a garnish. Chop the chili pepper. Add aubergine to hot frying pan; cook until browned, about 4 minutes, stirring frequently. Add oil, then chopped onion, pepper and garlic; cook 3 minutes, stirring occasionally. Add tomatoes and chopped chili pepper. Reduce heat; simmer uncovered 10 minutes, or until vegetables are tender and sauce thickens. Remove from heat; stir in salad greens and thyme. Season to taste with salt and pepper if desired. Drain pasta; transfer to two serving plates and top with sauce.

What's in it for you?

Total fat	4.3g	Carbohydrates	95.2g	Calcium	179mg
Saturated fat	0.6g	Sugar	15.4g	Magnesium	183mg
Healthy fats	2.9g	Protein	17.6g	Selenium	65.5mcg
Fibre	6.3g	Sodium	533mg	Potassium	1,163mg

Apricot Chicken and Fine Beans with Almond Slivers

2 servings • 430 calories per serving

Chicken Ingredients

2 skinless, boneless chicken breast halves (about 115g each) or
    substitute pork
4 dried apricots, chopped
2 tablespoons white wine
2 shallots, chopped
1 tablespoon olive oil
⅛ teaspoon ground cinnamon

Green Bean Ingredients

85g fine green beans
3 shallots, thinly sliced
1 tablespoon olive oil
1 teaspoon wine vinegar
1 teaspoon maple syrup
30g slivered almonds
Salt and freshly ground black pepper (optional)

To make the chicken, heat oven to 375°F/190°C/GM5. Place chicken in a glass baking dish. Sauté remaining chicken ingredients together until tender; transfer to blender or food processor and purée. Spoon over chicken and bake until chicken is cooked through, 15 to 20 minutes. Meanwhile, to prepare the beans, steam or blanch beans until tender but still firm and bright green. Sauté shallots in olive oil, vinegar and maple syrup until translucent. Add almonds and brown slightly; toss with beans. Season to taste with salt and pepper if desired. Serve alongside chicken.

What's in it for you?

Total fat	22g	Carbohydrates	25g	Calcium	95mg
Saturated fat	2.8g	Sugar	3.5g	Magnesium	100mg
Healthy fats	18.1g	Protein	32.7g	Selenium	22.4mcg
Fibre	4.6g	Sodium	89mg	Potassium	813mg

Turkey Tortilla Wraps with Red Baked Potato

2 servings • 497 calories per serving

Red Potato Ingredients

1 large russet baking potato, washed, pierced with tip of knife

2 tablespoons marinara sauce or other red tomato sauce

Turkey Wrap Ingredients

Two 6-inch wholewheat flour tortillas

4 slices roast turkey breast

4 romaine lettuce leaves

4 slices tomato

2 thin slices red or yellow onion

Mustard or hot peppers (optional)

To make the red potato, cook in microwave on high power
8 to 9 minutes or until fork-tender. Slice lengthwise in half;
spoon 1 tablespoon sauce over each half. Meanwhile, to
prepare the turkey wraps, layer all turkey wrap ingredients
on tortillas; roll up.

What's in it for you?

Total fat	14.5g	Carbohydrates	64g	Calcium	180mg
Saturated fat	4.5g	Sugar	6.5g	Magnesium	71mg
Healthy fats	10g	Protein	28.5g	Selenium	11.3mcg
Fibre	7g	Sodium	1,654mg	Potassium	1,596mg

Chicken Kebabs with Tabbouleh

2 servings • 397 calories per serving

Chicken Ingredients

2 skinless, boneless chicken breast halves (about 115g each),
    cut into 1-inch cubes

1 teaspoon dried oregano

½ teaspoon dried sage

1 red chili pepper, crushed (optional)

1 onion, quartered

1 tomato, quartered

1 pepper, seeded, stemmed, quartered

4 button mushrooms

Tabbouleh Ingredients

115g bulgur wheat

340ml boiling water

1 tomato, chopped

1 bunch green onions, chopped

1 large bunch parsley, finely chopped

1 small bunch fresh mint leaves, finely chopped

2 tablespoons lemon juice

1 tablespoon olive oil

Salt and freshly ground black pepper (optional)

Toss chicken with oregano, sage and, if desired, chili pepper. Alternately thread chicken, onion, tomato, pepper and mushrooms onto metal skewers. Cook under a preheated grill for 3 to 4 minutes per side, or until chicken is cooked through and vegetables are tender. Meanwhile, to prepare the tabbouleh, place bulgur wheat in medium bowl; add boiling water and mix well. Let stand until all water is absorbed, about 30 minutes. (Pour off any excess water.) Add remaining ingredients except salt and pepper; mix well. Season with salt and pepper if desired. Serve tabbouleh with grilled chicken and vegetables.

What's in it for you?

Total fat	9.4g	Carbohydrates	72.1g	Calcium	93mg
Saturated fat	1.5g	Sugar	12.1g	Magnesium	148mg
Healthy fats	7.1g	Protein	14.2g	Selenium	68mcg
Fibre	5.6g	Sodium	22.4mg	Potassium	1,121mg

Lemon Caper Chicken with Sweet Potato Purée

2 servings • 273 calories per serving

Chicken Ingredients

2 skinless, boneless chicken thighs (about 115g each)

Juice of 1 lemon

1 tablespoon olive oil

2 shallots, grated

1 tablespoon capers, drained

1 teaspoon Dijon mustard

Sweet Potato Ingredients

2 sweet potatoes, microwaved or baked

2 tablespoons orange juice

30g sultanas

½ teaspoon ground cinnamon

Salt and freshly ground black pepper (optional)

To make the chicken, preheat grill. Place chicken in a shallow roasting pan. Combine remaining chicken ingredients and pour over chicken. Cook 6 inches from heat source 12 to 15 minutes, or until chicken is cooked through. To prepare the potatoes, scoop hot sweet potato pulp into bowl. Add remaining sweet potato ingredients except salt and pepper; mix well. Season to taste with salt and pepper if desired. Serve with chicken.

What's in it for you?

Total fat	10.9g	Carbohydrates	20.6g	Calcium	39.5mg
Saturated fat	2g	Sugar	12.7g	Magnesium	41mg
Healthy fats	7.9g	Protein	24.7g	Selenium	16.5mcg
Fibre	1.4g	Sodium	336mg	Potassium	494mg

Grilled Trout with Rosemary and Lemon

2 servings • 182 calories per serving

225g whole trout
Salt and freshly ground black pepper (optional)
2 garlic cloves, sliced
4 sprigs of fresh rosemary
1 lemon, sliced

Preheat grill. Open fish like a book; season to taste with salt and pepper if desired. Arrange garlic, rosemary and lemon slices on one side of each fish; close other side and transfer fish to greased grill rack. Grill 5 to 6 inches from heat source 5 minutes. Turn fish over; continue to cook 4 to 5 minutes, or until fish is opaque throughout.

What's in it for you?

Total fat	7.3g	Carbohydrates	10.3g	Calcium	76mg
Saturated fat	1g	Sugar	4.9g	Magnesium	43mg
Healthy fat	4.9g	Protein	15.8g	Selenium	10.7mcg
Fibre	2.7g	Sodium	126mg	Potassium	688mg

Hot Wild Salmon

2 servings • 384 calories per serving

2 wild salmon fillets with skin (about 115g each) or salmon
    steaks (preferably line-caught)
2 tablespoons finely chopped fresh ginger
1 tablespoon wasabi paste
¼ teaspoon turmeric
Rock Asparagus (recipe on page 333)

Preheat grill. Brush skinless side of salmon with combined
ginger, wasabi paste and turmeric. Grill 4 to 6 inches from
heat source 10 to 12 minutes without turning, or until
salmon is opaque in centre. Serve with Rock Asparagus.

What's in it for you?

Total fat	14.5g	Carbohydrates	2.7g	Calcium	31mg
Saturated fat	2.3g	Sugar	0.2g	Magnesium	73mg
Healthy fats	10.6g	Protein	45.2g	Selenium	82.5mcg
Fibre	0.4g	Sodium	11mg	Potassium	1,176mcg

Grilled Peanut Prawns with Sesame Mangetout

2 servings • 163 calories per serving

Peanut Sauce Ingredients

1 tablespoon chunky peanut butter

1 tablespoon tinned light coconut milk

1 teaspoon fresh lime juice

Pinch of cayenne pepper

1 teaspoon honey

¼ teaspoon soy sauce

60ml water

1 garlic clove, peeled

10 medium uncooked prawns, peeled and deveined

Mangetout Ingredients

115g fresh mangetout

1 garlic clove, grated

1 teaspoon sesame seeds

1 teaspoon olive oil

½ teaspoon toasted sesame oil

Preheat grill. Place all ingredients for peanut sauce except prawns in blender or food processor; purée. Pour mixture over prawns; let stand 15 minutes. Thread prawns onto skewers; discard any excess marinade not clinging to prawns. Grill 2 to 3 minutes per side, or until prawns are opaque. Meanwhile, blanch mangetout in boiling water 2 minutes; drain and rinse with cold water. Cook garlic and sesame seeds in olive and sesame oils 2 minutes. Add drained mangetout; heat through, tossing well. Serve with prawns.

What's in it for you?

Total fat	10.5g	Carbohydrates	8.8g	Calcium	51.5mg
Saturated fat	2.9g	Sugar	5.1g	Magnesium	40.6mg
Healthy fats	7g	Protein	9.5g	Selenium	13.1mcg
Fibre	1.9g	Sodium	128mg	Potassium	220mg

Vegetable Tofu Stir-fry

2 servings • 602 calories per serving

1 tablespoon olive oil

½ teaspoon toasted sesame oil

¼ teaspoon crushed red pepper flakes

½ onion, sliced

2 garlic cloves, sliced

55g broccoli florets

½ red pepper, sliced

6 large button mushrooms, halved

1 teaspoon soy sauce

4 small 55g blocks baked tofu, cubed

2 green onions, chopped

1 small bunch coriander, chopped

1 teaspoon sesame seeds

In wok or large skillet, heat olive and sesame oils and pepper flakes over medium-high heat. Add onion and garlic; stir-fry 2 minutes. Add broccoli, pepper, mushrooms and soy sauce; stir-fry until vegetables are crisp-tender, 2 to 3 minutes. Add tofu, green onions, coriander and sesame seeds; stir-fry until heated through.

What's in it for you?

Total fat	23g	Carbohydrates	43g	Calcium	400mg
Saturated fat	3.3g	Sugar	16.4g	Magnesium	273mg
Healthy fats	18.9g	Protein	62.2g	Selenium	13.5mcg
Fibre	11.1g	Sodium	873mg	Potassium	2,403mg

Tofu or Turkey Dogs with Sauerkraut

2 Servings • 298 calories per serving

4 tofu (meatless) or turkey hot dogs
85g sauerkraut
Wholewheat buns (optional)
2 tablespoons favourite mustard, such as spicy brown or
    coarse-grained

Simmer hot dogs in water with sauerkraut until heated
through, about 5 minutes. Drain; serve with mustard (with
or without buns).

What's in it for you?

Total fat	26g	Carbohydrates	3.8g	Calcium	158mg
Saturated fat	9g	Sugar	2.1g	Magnesium	27mg
Healthy fats	15.4g	Protein	11.2g	Selenium	1.9mcg
Fibre	0.7g	Sodium	1,219mg	Potassium	160mg

YOU Side Dishes

Rock Asparagus

4 servings • 38 calories per serving

455g asparagus spears, rinsed, dried and trimmed
1 teaspoon extra-virgin olive oil
Sea salt, to taste (optional)
¼ teaspoon *each*: dried thyme, oregano, basil and black
    pepper
Optional garnish: diced tomato

Heat oven to 350°F/180°C/GM4. Toss the asparagus in a
13 x 9-inch baking dish or a shallow casserole pan with the
olive oil, salt if desired, thyme, oregano, basil and black
pepper. Arrange asparagus in a single layer in the dish.
Bake uncovered 12 to 13 minutes for thin asparagus or 15
to 18 minutes for thick asparagus, or until crisp-tender.
Garnish with tomato if desired.

What's in it for you?

Total fat	1.5g	Carbohydrates	5g	Calcium	27mg
Saturated fat	0.2g	Sugar	1.8g	Magnesium	22mg
Healthy fats	1.1g	Protein	2.9g	Selenium	4mcg
Fibre	1.4g	Sodium	5mg	Potassium	352mg

Tomato-avocado Salsamole

2 servings • 90 calories per serving

30g finely chopped red onion

1 teaspoon grated jalapeño, or more to taste

1 tablespoon lime juice

1 tablespoon cider vinegar

1 teaspoon grated garlic

¼ teaspoon salt

1 ripe avocado, peeled, pitted and coarsely mashed

1 medium tomato, chopped

¼ teaspoon chopped coriander

Combine onion, jalapeño, lime juice, vinegar, garlic and salt in bowl. Add avocado, tomato and coriander; stir well. Serve immediately or, to store, reserve avocado stone, add to mixture to prevent browning, cover tightly with cling film and refrigerate. Serve with lightly toasted wholewheat pitta cut into triangles.

What's in it for you?

Total fat	8g	Carbohydrates	8g	Calcium	20mg
Saturated fat	2.1g	Sugar	2g	Magnesium	54mg
Healthy fats	5.3g	Protein	2g	Selenium	0mcg
Fibre	3.1g	Sodium	25mg	Potassium	805mg

YOU Desserts

Cinnamon Baked Apples with Tangerines and Cranberries

4 servings • 146 calories per serving

2 large baking apples (or substitute pears)
285ml unsweetened apple juice, preferably unfiltered organic
55g dried cranberries (or substitute cherries)
¼ teaspoon ground cinnamon
¼ teaspoon ground cloves
2 seedless clementines or tangerines, peeled, separated into
     segments

Heat oven to 400°F/200°C/GM6. Cut apples in half lengthwise; cut out and discard cores, seeds and stems. Place 60ml of the apple juice in an 8-inch baking dish or casserole pan. Place apples cut side down on juice. Bake 15 to 18 minutes or until apples are tender. Meanwhile, simmer remaining apple juice in a small saucepan over medium-high heat 5 minutes. Add cranberries, cinnamon and cloves; reduce heat and simmer uncovered 10 minutes, or until cranberries are plumped, stirring occasionally. Remove from heat; stir in clementine sections. Arrange apple halves cut side up on serving dishes. Pour any remaining liquid from dish into cranberry mixture; spoon over apples.

What's in it for you?

Total fat	0.6g	Carbohydrates	37.7g	Calcium	30mg
Saturated fat	0.1g	Sugar	30.4g	Magnesium	13mg
Healthy fats	0.3g	Protein	0.7g	Zinc	0.1mg
Fibre	4.1g	Sodium	15mg	Selenium	0.2mg
				Potassium	281mg

Cinnamon Apple Sauté à la Mode

2 servings • 220 calories per serving

2 small apples
1 tablespoon apple butter
1 tablespoon unsweetened apple juice or cider, preferably
    organic
½ teaspoon ground cinnamon
6 walnut halves, toasted, coarsely chopped
115g fat-free or low-fat vanilla frozen yogurt

Cut apples into quarters; discard stems, cores and seeds.
Cut apple quarters into thin slices. Heat a large nonstick
frying pan over medium-high heat until hot. Add apples;
cook until apples begin to brown, about 4 minutes, tossing occasionally. Stir in apple butter, apple juice and cinnamon; continue to cook 5 to 8 minutes, or until apples are
tender and sauce thickens, tossing frequently. Transfer to
serving plates; top with nuts. Serve with frozen yogurt.

What's in it for you?

Total fat	8.4g	Carbohydrates	38g	Calcium	83mg
Saturated fat	0.8g	Sugar	27.6g	Magnesium	35mg
Healthy fats	7.0g	Protein	3.6g	Selenium	2mcg
Fibre	6.7g	Sodium	23mg	Potassium	346mg

Sliced Peaches with Raspberries, Blueberries and Chocolate Chips

2 servings • 46 calories per serving

2 small ripe peaches, sliced
½ teaspoon ground cinnamon
Pinch of nutmeg
30g fresh raspberries
30g fresh blueberries
1½ tablespoons mini semi-sweet chocolate chips

Combine sliced peaches with cinnamon and nutmeg; transfer to two serving plates. Top peaches with raspberries, blueberries and chocolate chips.

What's in it for you?

Total fat	0.4g	Carbohydrates	11.5g	Calcium	22mg
Saturated fat	0.1g	Sugar	8.9g	Magnesium	11.5mg
Healthy fats	0.28g	Protein	1g	Selenium	0.1mcg
Fibre	2.6g	Sodium	0.5mg	Potassium	202mg

Roasted Pear with Raspberry Coulis, Chocolate and Pistachios

2 servings • 184 calories per serving

1 large red pear

115ml white wine (high-quality)

6oz frozen unsweetened raspberries, thawed, or 115g fresh
    raspberries

1 tablespoon mini semi-sweet chocolate chips

1½ tablespoons coarsely chopped pistachios, toasted

Heat oven to 400°F/200°F/GM6. Cut pear in half; remove
core with a melon baller or metal teaspoon. Arrange pear
halves, cut side down, in a shallow baking dish. Pour wine
over pears. Bake 18 to 20 minutes, or until pears are
tender when pierced with the tip of a sharp knife. Meanwhile, purée raspberries in food processor; strain and
discard seeds. Transfer roasted pears to serving plates, cut
side up; sprinkle chocolate chips over the pears (the heat
of the pears will melt the chips). Combine puréed raspberries and liquid remaining in baking dish in a small
saucepan. Cook over high heat until sauce is slightly thick-
ened. Spoon sauce over and around pears; sprinkle with
pistachios. Serve warm or at room temperature.

What's in it for you?

Total fat	5.2g	Carbohydrates	31.8g	Calcium	45mg
Saturated fat	1.4g	Sugar	24g	Magnesium	32mg
Healthy fats	3.3g	Protein	2.7g	Selenium	2mcg
Fibre	4.9g	Sodium	7mg	Potassium	344mg

YOU Snack

Simon's Popcorn

4 servings • 61 calories per serving, 10 per cent from fat

85g popcorn kernels
Flavoured cooking spray (butter, olive oil or garlic)
Garlic salt or cinnamon

Place popcorn in a deep, large microwave-safe container; cover and cook at high power 4 to 5 minutes, or until popcorn is popped but not scorched. If the microwave oven does not have a rotating turntable, use oven mitts to grasp and shake the covered container after 3 minutes of cooking. Immediately pour the popcorn onto a baking sheet and coat with cooking spray. To further flavour the popcorn, immediately sprinkle on your favourite seasoning blend such as garlic salt or cinnamon.

What's in it for you?

Total fat	0.8g	Carbohydrates	5g	Calcium	1mg
Saturated fat	0.1g	Sugar	0g	Magnesium	0mg
Healthy fats	0.7g	Protein	1g	Selenium	1mcg
Fibre	0.4g	Sodium	0mg	Potassium	0mg

INDEX